GARBHKATHA

21 Tales Unlocking Vedic Secrets of Manifesting Dream Child

PAYAL MEHTA

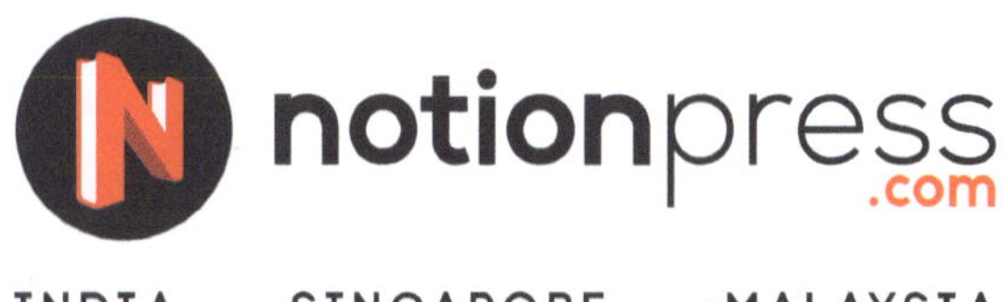

INDIA • SINGAPORE • MALAYSIA

ISBN
Hardcase 979-8-89632-736-3
Paperback 979-8-89446-606-4

Dedicated

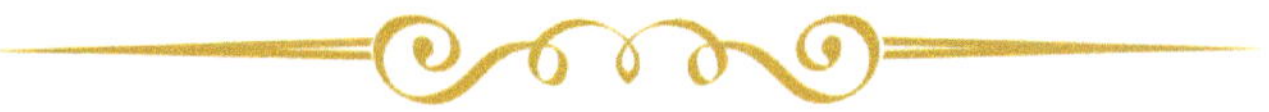

To my beautiful daughter, Kiyara,
Whose mere presence inspired me to write this book.
Thanks, Kiyara, for bringing consistency, persistence, and discipline into my life.

Contents

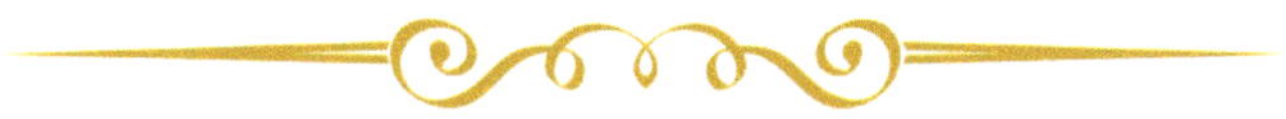

Contents

Acknowledgement

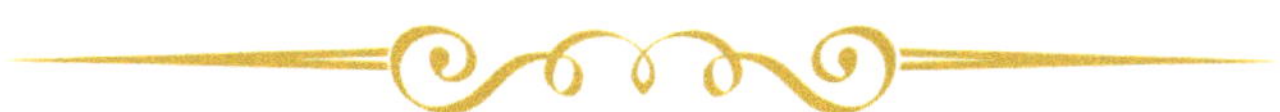

Writing a book is not an easy endeavour; it demands you to pour your heart, mind, and soul into every page. You must navigate through self-doubt, procrastination, fear, and countless distractions to see it through to completion. Writing a book had always been on my mind, but I couldn't commit to it until I became a mother. Looking after a newborn, managing my IT job, researching, and writing late at night was incredibly tough yet exhilarating, enchanting but insane, and gratifying but draining. And without the support of my loved ones, I couldn't have done it.

I owe a special debt of thanks to my mother, Revati Mehta, whose suggestions were indispensable for this project.

Special thanks to my dad, Shirish Mehta, for always encouraging me to expand my horizons.

I am grateful to my husband, my heartthrob Vipul Shah, for his unwavering support in all my ventures, no matter how crazy they sound.

I deeply appreciate the efforts of my mother-in-law, Padmashree Shah, for taking care of all household duties and making it possible for me to pursue my passion alongside a successful IT career.

I would also like to mention Dr. Pallavi Desai and Dr. Prajkta Gawde, both women of exceptional insight and talent, for their wise counsel. Finally, I would like to thank all the parents who are part of the "Srujan Scientific GarbhaSanksar" family and who trusted me enough to share their feelings and experiences.

Preface

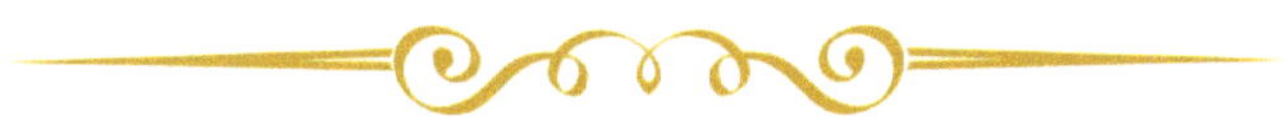

I've always been captivated by the mysteries of babies—why some are serene while others seem to wail at every turn, why some eagerly devour every bite while others turn their noses up at food, and why some reach developmental milestones with ease while others take their time. This curiosity turned into a deep obsession when I began considering having a child of my own. I wanted to find a way to guarantee the whole health—physical, mental, emotional, social, and spiritual—of my unborn child. My research led me to the concept of GarbhSanskar, which combines "Garbha," meaning womb, with "Sanskar," meaning education. Educating an unborn child in the womb, as an engineer with a logical mindset, I was initially sceptical. However, after extensive research and finding scientific backing, I became convinced of its validity. I was surprised to see many people being unaware of this ancient Vedic practice and decided to promote it through webinars and workshops. Seeing the positive results in parents who practised GarbhSanskar boosted my confidence immensely.

When I became pregnant, I adhered to the principles of GarbhSanskar and experienced remarkable results. The journey of integrating these practices into my daily life was transformative, not just for my baby but for me as well. I noticed profound changes in my own emotional and mental well-being, which positively influenced my pregnancy experience. The birth of my daughter, Kiyara, was the most profound moment of my life. Though she was born a month earlier, she weighed a healthy 3.4 kg and did not look like a premature baby from any angle. She achieved all her milestones before time. At just

2 years old, she could sit and focus for 30 minutes straight, which helped her become the fastest toddler to solve a Montessori puzzle, earning a prestigious record in the India Book of Records. Since childhood, she has been obsessed with books. Her healthy body, sound mind, sharp intellect, emotional quotient, and spiritual nature are byproducts of GarbhSanskar practices followed during pregnancy. After experiencing the miracles of GarbhSanskar myself, I want to spread this awareness to enable future parents to take advantage of this age-old wisdom. Through this book, I wish to inspire planning and pregnant couples to follow GarbhSanskar during pregnancy.

This Being my first book, holds a special place in my heart. Writing it has been more than a creative endeavour—it has been a journey of profound personal transformation. As I brought my thoughts and ideas to life on the page, I uncovered parts of myself I never knew existed. Every word and chapter became a mirror, reflecting my experiences, emotions, and growth.

This journey challenged me to confront my fears and insecurities, pushing me to explore my deepest thoughts and beliefs. It became an adventure of self-discovery, reshaping my perspective on life and my role within it. GarbhKatha is not just a collection of stories or ideas; it stands as a testament to the evolution of my identity and a milestone in my personal development.

Foreword

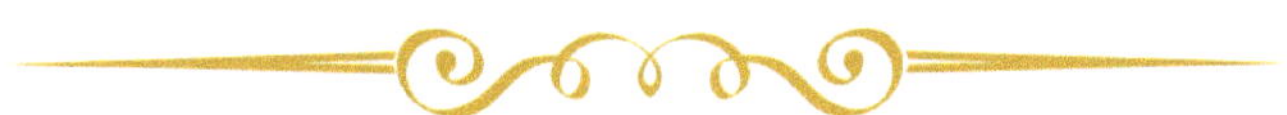

The journey of parenthood begins well before a child's birth. Ancient Vedic philosophy emphasizes that a mother's thoughts, emotions, and actions profoundly influence the consciousness of her unborn child. This understanding forms the essence of GarbhSanskar, an age-old practice that fosters the mental, emotional, and spiritual well-being of a child during pregnancy.

Deeply rooted in Indian culture, GarbhSanskar refers to the practice of nurturing and educating a child even in the womb. It highlights the importance of holistic development, starting from conception, rather than waiting until after birth. Today, with advancements in psychology and medicine, the value of prenatal education is increasingly recognized, aligning modern science with ancient wisdom. GarbhSanskar is not merely a cultural tradition but a scientifically supported approach to shaping the physical, mental, emotional, social, and spiritual growth of an unborn child.

In GarbhKatah - 21 Tales Unlocking Vedic Secrets of Having a Dream Child, Payal Mehta beautifully blends ancient wisdom, mythology, history, and modern science to guide expectant parents. Through 21 captivating stories, this book reveals the profound connection between a mother's state of mind and her child's development, offering lessons that remain relevant in today's world. Each story educates and inspires, presenting Vedic concepts in an accessible and relatable manner. Drawing from mythology, historical figures, and modern-day examples, Payal paints a vivid picture of the transformative power of mindfulness, intention, and positive conditioning during pregnancy.

This book serves as a roadmap for parents seeking to welcome a child with love, awareness, and wisdom. Payal's perspective—as a software engineer, a GarbhSanskar coach and a mother who has experienced the impact of these practices firsthand—adds authenticity and depth to her work. Her journey exemplifies the possibilities that arise when ancient traditions meet modern understanding.

I am mesmerized by this author and mother, Payal Mehta, who is excelling in her IT career, leading teams in a high-tech company, is very modern and yet wholeheartedly embracing and promoting traditional values, staying deeply rooted in her culture. We need more mothers who exemplify this remarkable balance. May these stories deepen your understanding of the unseen influences that shape a child's destiny before birth.

With reverence and gratitude,
Baba Naikade (Retd IFS)
Famous Pravachankar – spiritual Guru,
M.A. Marathi, M.A. Philosophy,
M.Sc (Agri), M.Sc (Forestry),
LLB, DLL & LW, ADCSSA

Introduction

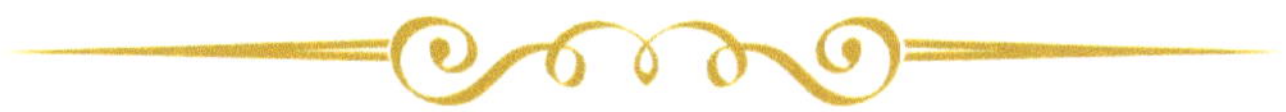

Welcome to **GarbhKatha**, a collection that delves into the profound and transformative journey of pregnancy. As you turn these pages, you will discover 21 stories that beautifully intertwine the science, spirituality, and awe of bringing new life into the world.

The title "GarbhKatha" is a blend of ancient wisdom and modern understanding. "Garbh," derived from Sanskrit, refers to the womb—the sacred space where life begins. "Katha" means story or narrative, encapsulating the essence of our shared human experience. Together, they embody the narrative of pregnancy—a journey that is as much about the physical experience as it is about the emotional and spiritual transformations that occur. Each story reveals unique insights and secrets to nurturing not just a healthy baby, but a child of virtue and strength. These insights are decoded from the ancient Vedic practice of **GarbhSanskar**, which emphasises the importance of nurturing a child's potential even before birth. The enchanting tales presented in this collection blend practical advice, personal reflections, and timeless wisdom, highlighting the profound connection between parent and child. They reveal the significant impact that nurturing can have from the very start, shaping not just the child's physical health but also their character and future.

I invite you to explore these stories with an open heart and mind. Whether you are planning a child, expecting a child, or simply curious about the profound journey of pregnancy, **GarbhKatha** offers valuable insights and heartfelt stories that will resonate with you. May the stories within these pages illuminate your path and enrich your understanding of one of life's most remarkable adventures.

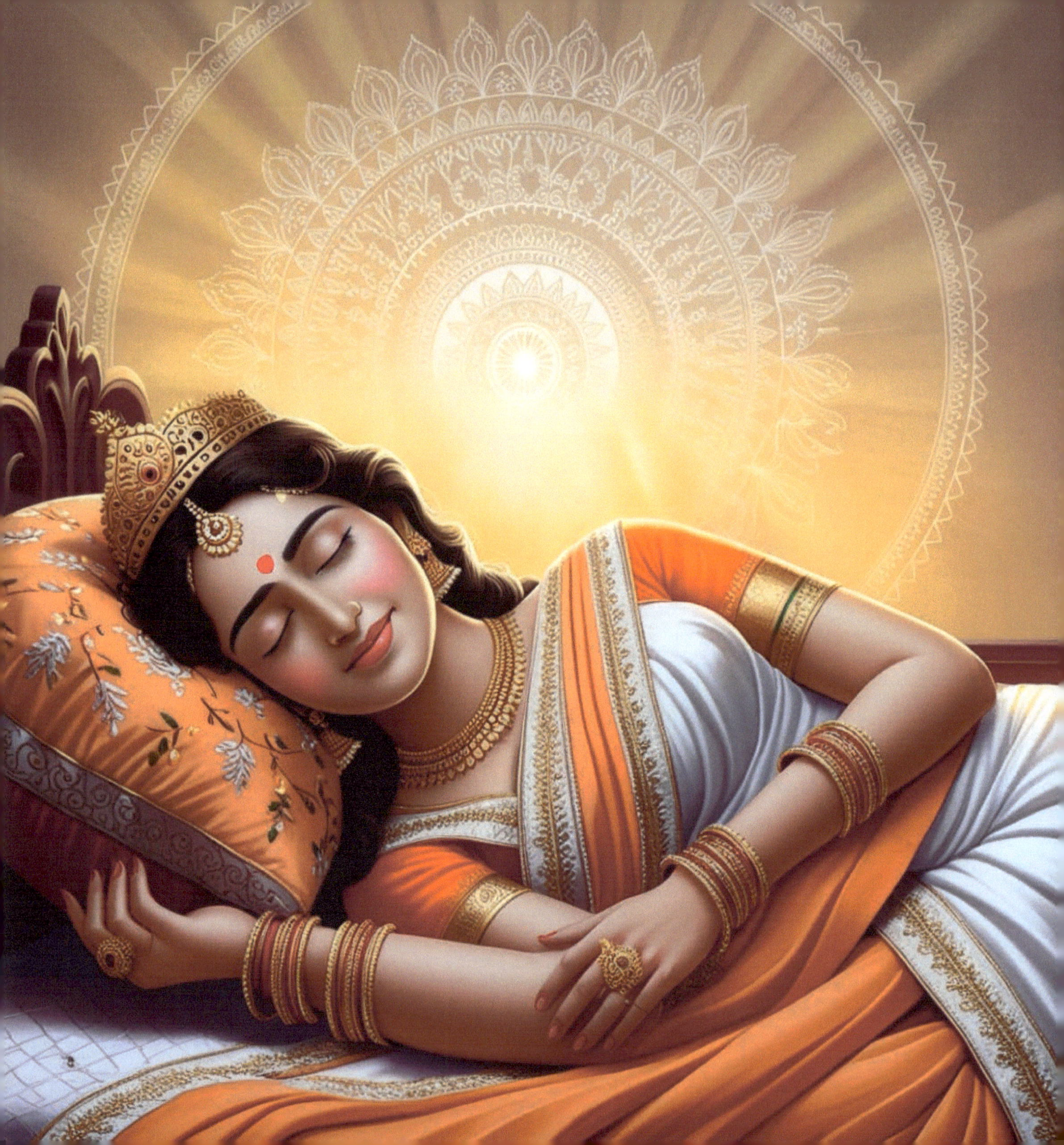

1. Echoes of Emotion

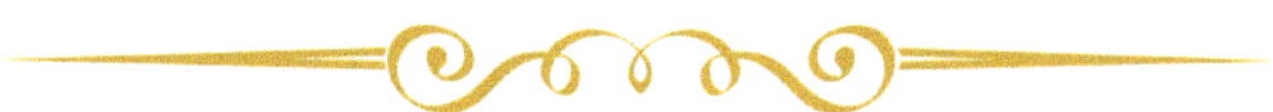

In the ancient kingdom of Vaishali, a land known for its wisdom and prosperity, lived a noble princess named Trishala, the eldest daughter of King Chetak. Her sharp intellect and deep compassion complemented her beauty and grace, which won the affection of all her subjects. Upon reaching adulthood, she was married to King Siddharth of Kundgraam, a union that was celebrated across the realms.

Queen Trishala experienced 16 auspicious dreams filled with miraculous visions while she was expecting Lord Mahaveera. Each dream promised a son who would be strong, brave, fearless, and capable of ruling the world. Visions foretold that the child would possess supreme knowledge and be endowed with boundless wisdom and virtues. He would liberate humanity from the cycle of birth, misery, and death. Recognising the significance of these dreams, Trishala's heart swelled with hope and pride.

Meanwhile, the bond between mother and child deepened in many ways unseen. While in the womb, Mahaveera sensed his mother's unease caused by his motions and instinctively paused his movements, wishing to soothe her. However, a reverse occurred. Trishala Mata became agitated and depressed. She even stopped eating assuming that the baby had died as there were no moments. The emotional turmoil of the mother did not escape Mahaveera's awareness, and he resumed his movements, filling her with relief and ecstatic joy.

After a few days, on the thirteenth day of the rising moon in the month of Chaitra, joy erupted in the royal palace as Vardhamana, the future Lord Mahaveera, was born.

King Siddhartha prospered immeasurably following his son's birth and named him Vardhamana, which means "increasing." He credited this newfound affluence and success to the arrival of his son.

As Vardhamana grew, he felt an undeniable calling for a higher purpose. At the age of 30, Vardhamana denounced his royal family life in pursuit of spiritual awakening. For the next 12 and a half years, he practised severe meditation and attained Keval Gyana. After achieving enlightenment, he shared his newfound knowledge with everyone in need. He spent the following 30 years touring India barefoot, spreading the crucial message of Ahimsa or non-violence. The term Ahimsa means non-violence, non-injury, and the absence of a desire to harm any life forms.

He condemned violence not only against humans but also against animals, plants, microorganisms, and all beings having life or life potential. His teachings inspired countless individuals to embrace Jainism, guiding them toward a life centred on non-violence and respect for all forms of life. Though he was the last Jain Tirthankara, his teachings and philosophies continue to resonate with people even today, illuminating paths towards compassion and understanding.

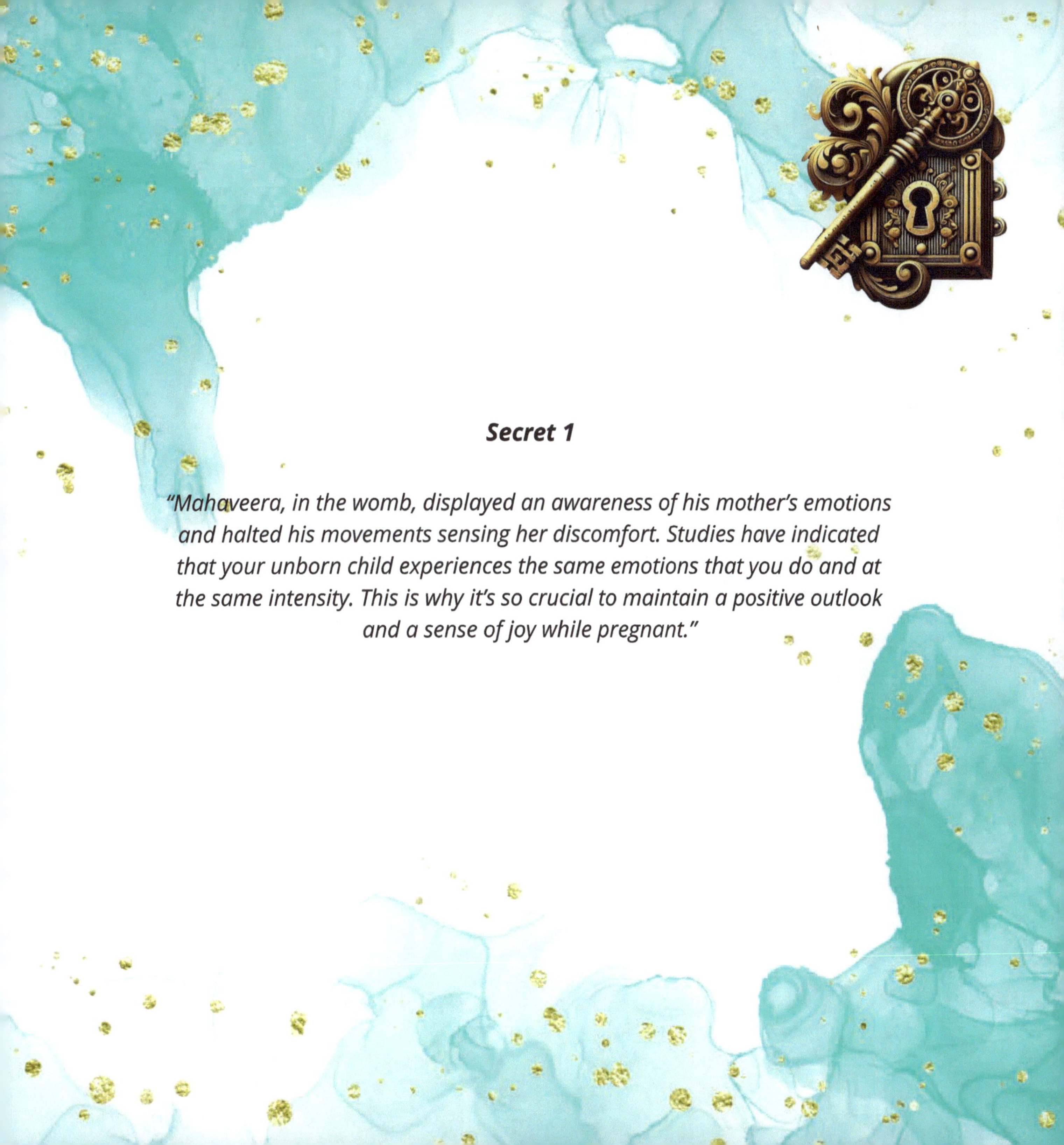

Secret 1

"Mahaveera, in the womb, displayed an awareness of his mother's emotions and halted his movements sensing her discomfort. Studies have indicated that your unborn child experiences the same emotions that you do and at the same intensity. This is why it's so crucial to maintain a positive outlook and a sense of joy while pregnant."

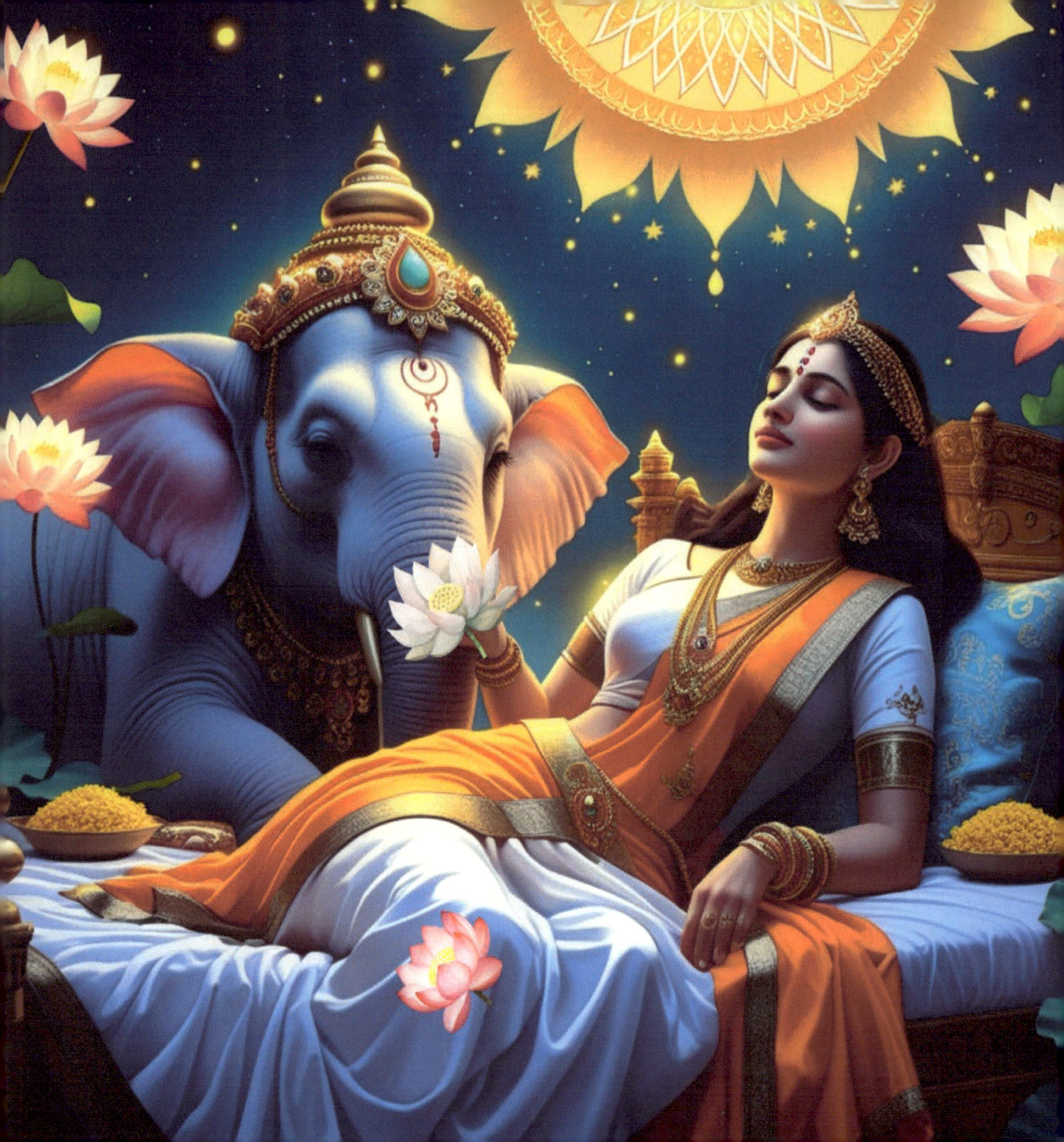

2. Nature of Nurturer

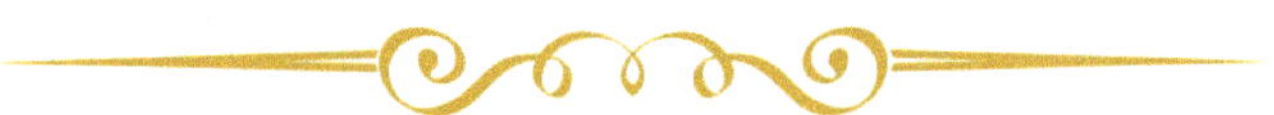

In the enchanting realms of the ancient Nepalese Devadaha dynasty, a remarkable princess named Mahamaya graced the world. Born to King Anjana and Queen Yasodhara, she embodied extraordinary beauty, intelligence, and virtue, captivating the hearts of all who knew her. When she reached marriageable age, she wed King Suddhodana of the Sakya clan. Known as the "King of the Law," Suddhodana was revered for his commitment to justice. He and Maya Devi complemented each other beautifully.

After 12 long years of marriage without a child, Queen Maya experienced a vivid and strange dream one full moon night. In her dream, she was lying on a celestial couch when a beautiful white baby elephant bearing a white lotus blossom in its trunk entered her womb. Upon interpreting the dream, the astrologers' proclaimed, "The child destined to be born is a soul of unparalleled purity, divinity, and holiness." Overjoyed by this prophecy, Maya and Suddhodana rejoiced.

Deeply spiritual by nature, Maya embraced the 5 precepts of morality during her pregnancy. She abstained from killing living beings, stealing, sexual misconduct, lying, and intoxication, striving to cultivate a life free of material attachment and greed. With her heart filled with love and devotion, she awaited the arrival of her child, enjoying a happy and healthy pregnancy. Although a typical pregnancy lasts 9 months, Queen Mahamaya's journey extended to 10 months. Finally, on one fine day in the serene Lumbini Garden, she gave birth to a baby boy whom they named "Siddharth".

As predicted by the Brahmins, Siddharth was destined to become either a monk or a "Chakravarti," a universal monarch. To steer him towards a life of rulership, King Suddhodana confined him within the opulent palace, surrounding him with every pleasure imaginable and shielding him from the harsh realities of life.

However, one day, driven by curiosity, Prince Siddharth slipped beyond the palace walls. He encountered an old man, a sick man, a dead man, and a religious ascetic. In that moment, he grasped the profound truths of existence—the inevitability of ageing, sickness, and death. This awakening compelled him to abandon worldly pleasures in search of enlightenment.

For 6 years, he wandered in pursuit of knowledge and understanding, immersing himself in meditation. Finally, at Bodhgaya, he resolved to remain in meditation until he uncovered the true nature of the mind. After spending 6 days and nights cutting through the most subtle obstacles of the mind, he attained enlightenment on the full moon morning of May, a week shy of his thirty-fifth birthday.

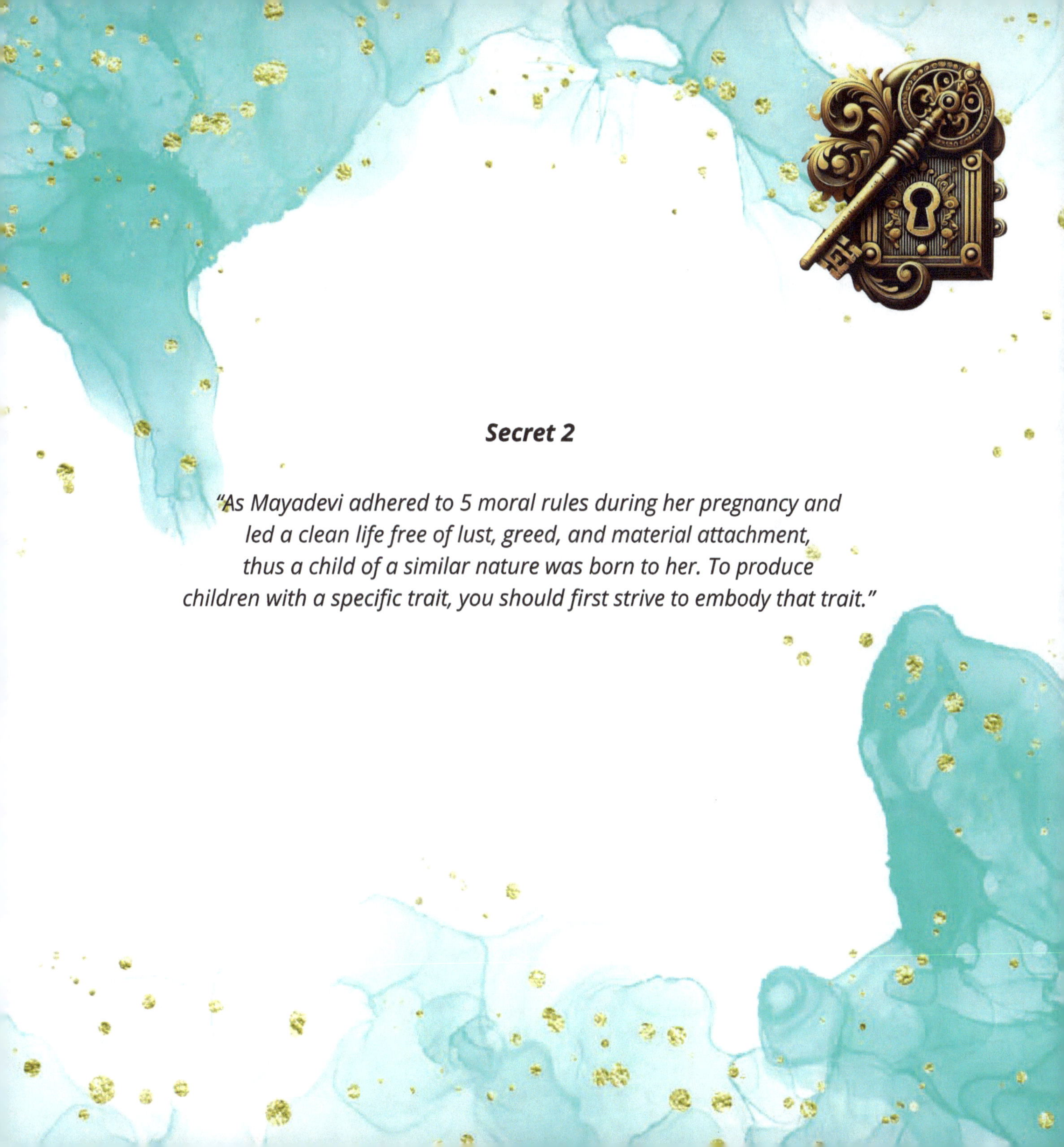

Secret 2

"As Mayadevi adhered to 5 moral rules during her pregnancy and led a clean life free of lust, greed, and material attachment, thus a child of a similar nature was born to her. To produce children with a specific trait, you should first strive to embody that trait."

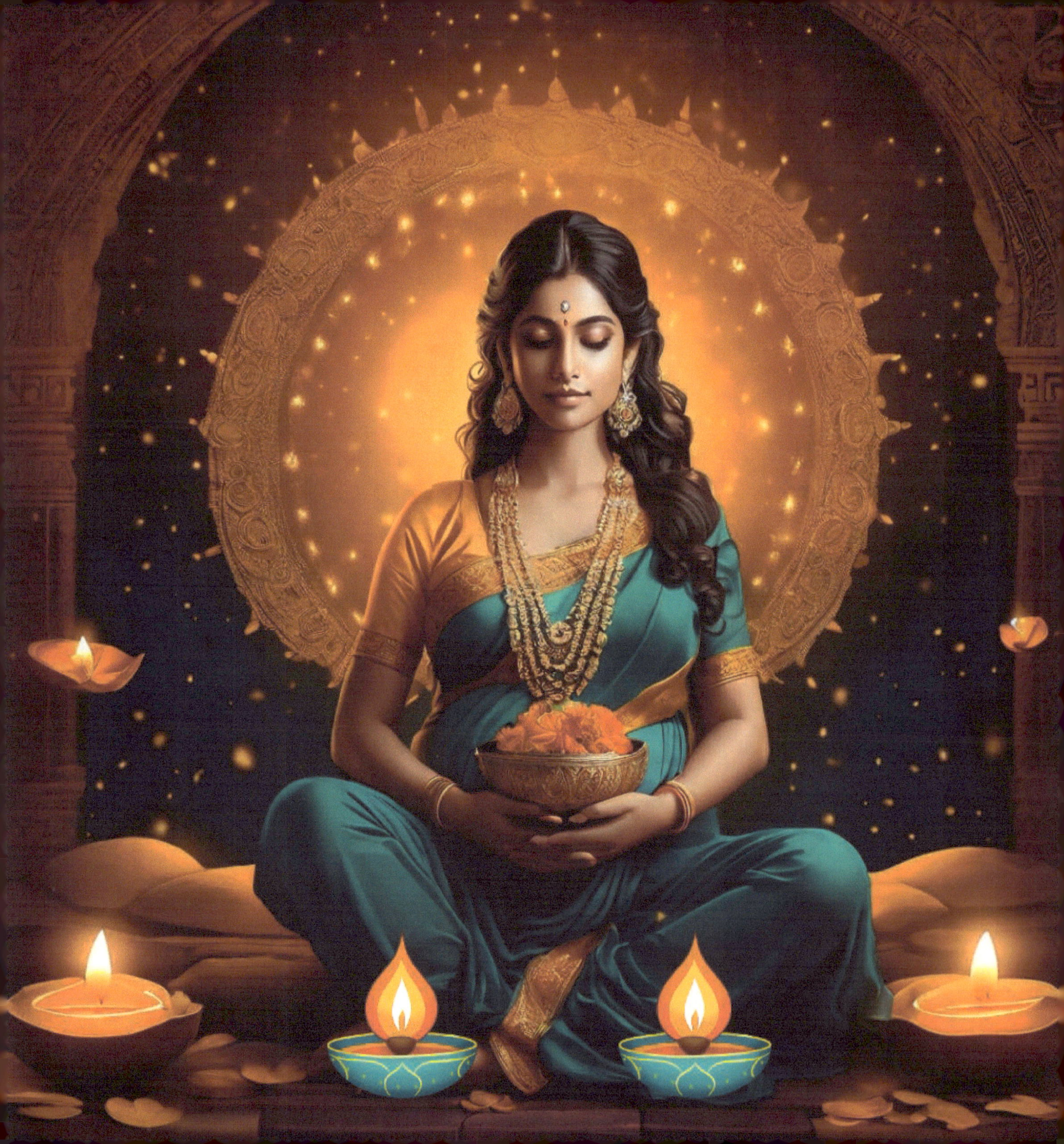

3. Power of Sanskara

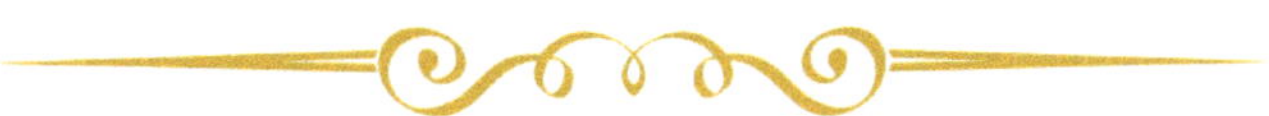

Kayadhu was the devoted wife of demon king Hiranyakashipu. Boastful, avaricious, and cruel, Hiranyakashipu harboured grand ambitions to conquer the world and to become the ruler of all 3 realms. Hiranyakashipu desired a boon from Brahma Deva which would almost make him immortal. For this reason, he left pregnant Kayadhu in the care of his prime minister, Vidal, and journeyed to the Himalayas to perform severe penance.

Indra, the King of the Gods, trembled at the thought of Hiranyakashipu receiving such power. Fearing that a granted boon would lead to his downfall, Indra invaded Hiranyakashipu's kingdom, abducting Kayadhu in a fit of desperation. In a dark moment, he attempted to harm her unborn child, but the divine sage Narada intervened, warning Indra that it would be a grave sin to harm the innocent.

Kayadhu was freed after that and taken to the tranquil ashrama of sage Narada, a place steeped in holiness. There, Sage Narada treated her like a daughter, showering her with motherly love and guidance. Addressing the unborn baby, he daily used to teach Kayadhu about the devotion one should have towards God. As directed by the sage Narada, Kayadhu would repeatedly recite the Narayana Mantra, "OM NAMO NARAYANAN NAMAHA." At such a young stage of development, the unborn child got sanskaras (morals and values) of devotion. In the sanctity of the ashrama, both mother and child became imbued with divine qualities, preparing the unborn Prahlada for a remarkable destiny.

When Hiranyakashipu returned from his penance, Narada respectfully handed over Kayadhu. The infant was eventually born and given the name Prahlada. Prahlada became a sincere devotee of Lord Vishnu as the sanskaras given by Narada were engraved on his mind, body, and soul. Hiranyakashipu tried to dissuade Prahlada from worshipping Vishnu. Despite several warnings, Prahlada did not stop. Enraged, Hiranyakashipu decided to punish him. He poisoned Prahlada, trampled the boy with elephants, put him in a room with venomous snakes, and threw him from a valley into a river, but he survived. One day he even tried to burn Prahlada alive with the help of his sister Holika but had no luck. Despite all these challenges, Prahlada followed the path of devotion fearlessly, courageously, and with utter sincerity.

Finally, Lord Narasimha, the half-man-half-lion avatar of Lord Vishnu, killed Hiranyakashipu as he was constantly abusing Prahlada. Following that, Prahlada took over his father's kingdom and ruled peacefully and virtuously. He was known for his generosity and kindness.

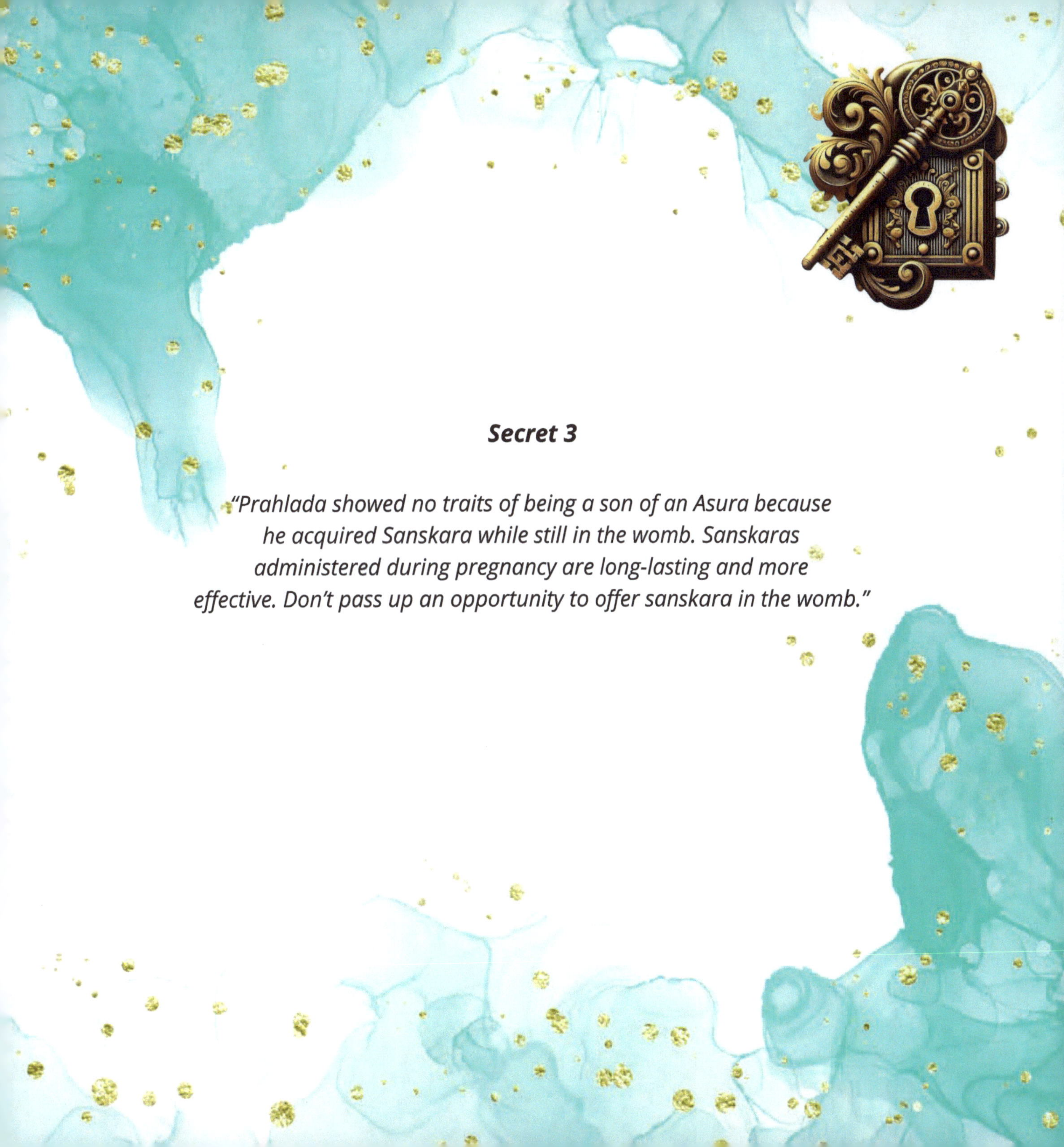

Secret 3

"Prahlada showed no traits of being a son of an Asura because he acquired Sanskara while still in the womb. Sanskaras administered during pregnancy are long-lasting and more effective. Don't pass up an opportunity to offer sanskara in the womb."

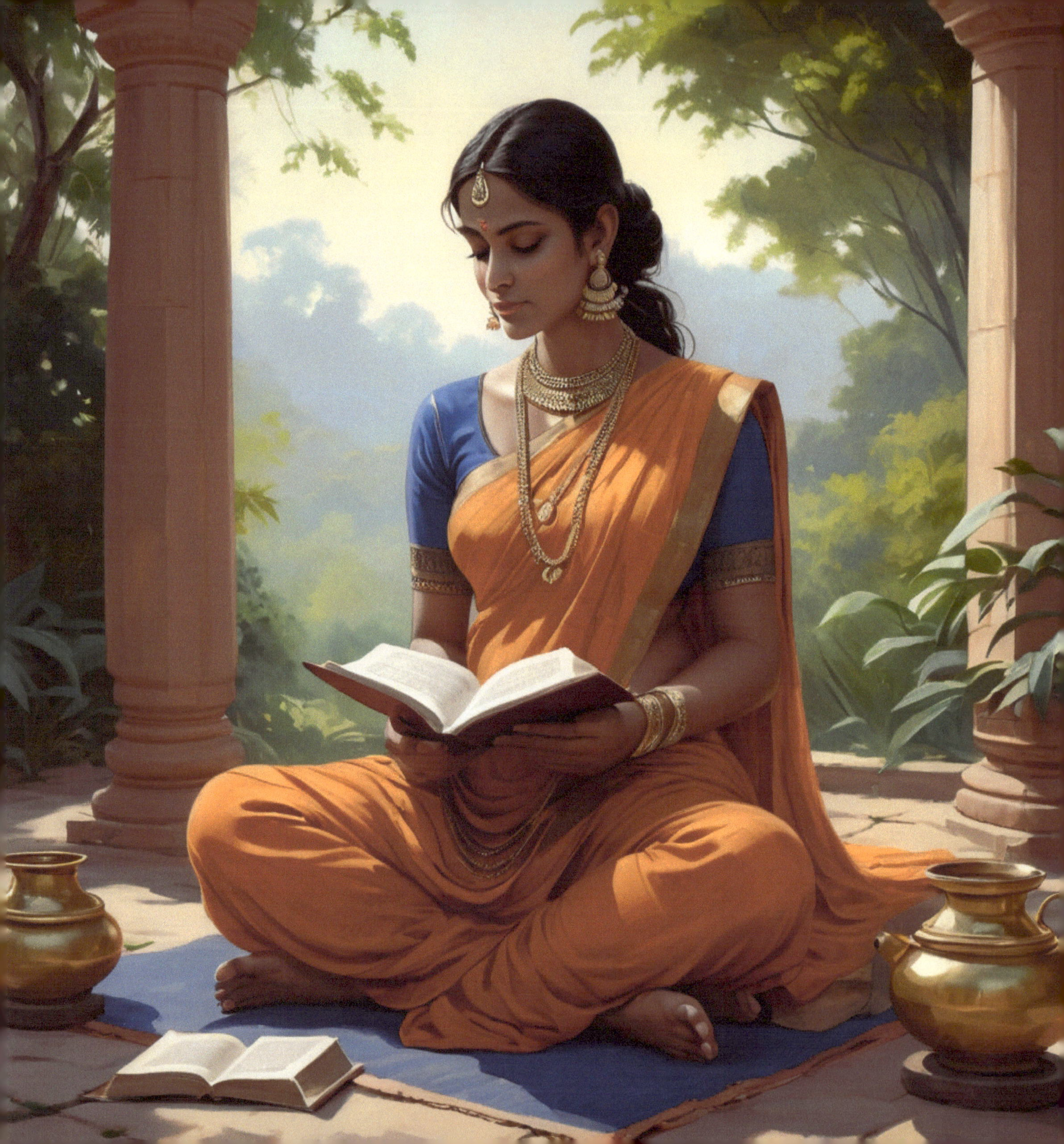

4. Born Brilliant

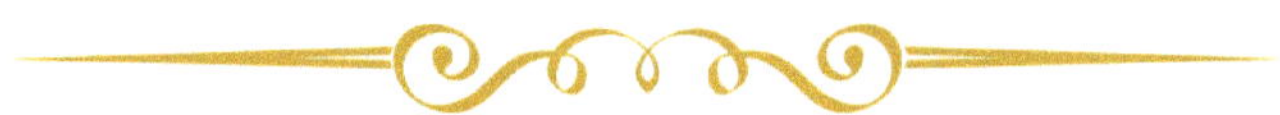

Sujata was the beloved daughter of the great sage Uddalaka Aruni. After completing his education with Guru Ayodh Daumya, Uddalaka established a Gurukul of his own. Known for his wisdom and patience, Uddalaka quickly became a respected teacher, attracting students from all corners of the land. Among these students was Kahoda, a humble but devoted learner. Though Kahoda initially struggled with the Scriptures and Vedas, his dedication and reverence for his teacher won Uddalaka's admiration.

When Sujata reached marriageable age, her father, impressed by Kahoda's devotion and sincerity, chose him as her husband. The union was a happy one, and Kahoda, inspired by Uddalaka's wisdom, began teaching alongside him in the Gurukul. Their life was peaceful, and soon, joy filled their hearts when Sujata discovered she was pregnant.

Overjoyed, Sujata longed for her child to be a brilliant scholar, one who would excel in knowledge of the Vedas and possess spiritual wisdom. With this desire in her heart, she began to attend her father's and husband's teachings, believing that the knowledge would reach her unborn child. Little did she know, her wish was coming true. The child within her, Ashtavakra, absorbed the teachings deeply and attained immense mastery over the Vedas and dimensions of the Self while still in the fetal state.

However, fate had other plans. One day, as Kahoda was reciting verses from the Vedas, he mispronounced a word. Each time he made a mistake, Sujata felt her child wiggle in the womb. On the eighth mistake, something remarkable happened—a small voice echoed from her womb, correcting the error with a firm "hum." The voice was clear and precise as if the child had already mastered the knowledge Kahoda was trying to impart.

Kahoda, though deeply committed to learning, was also a man of pride. Feeling humiliated by the correction, especially from his unborn child, his face darkened with anger. In a moment of frustration, he lashed out, "You arrogant child! How dare you correct me before you are even born? You've interrupted me 8 times! I curse you to be born deformed in 8 places, as a mark of your arrogance!"

Sujata gasped in horror, but the curse had been spoken. When the child was born, he emerged with bent limbs—his hands, feet, knees, chest, and neck were crooked. The child was named Ashtavakra, which means bends." Despite his physical deformities, Ashtavakra was no ordinary child. His intelligence and spiritual wisdom were evident from an early age.

Later, Ashtavakra defeats Bandi, son of God Varuna, in a debate organised by King Janaka. Kahoda, impressed by his son's wisdom, urged him to bathe in the sacred river Samanga, which miraculously healed all his abnormalities.

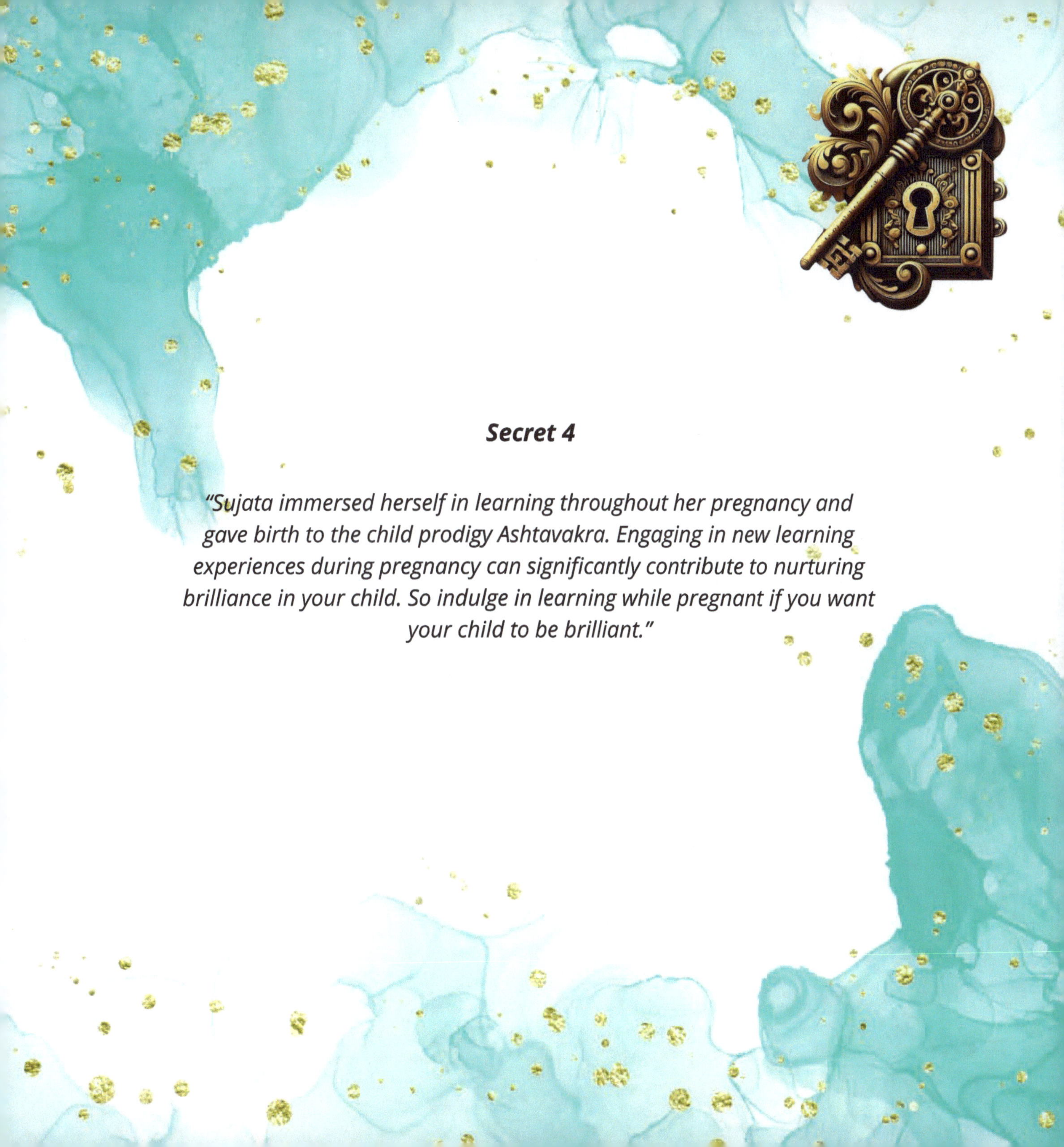

Secret 4

"Sujata immersed herself in learning throughout her pregnancy and gave birth to the child prodigy Ashtavakra. Engaging in new learning experiences during pregnancy can significantly contribute to nurturing brilliance in your child. So indulge in learning while pregnant if you want your child to be brilliant."

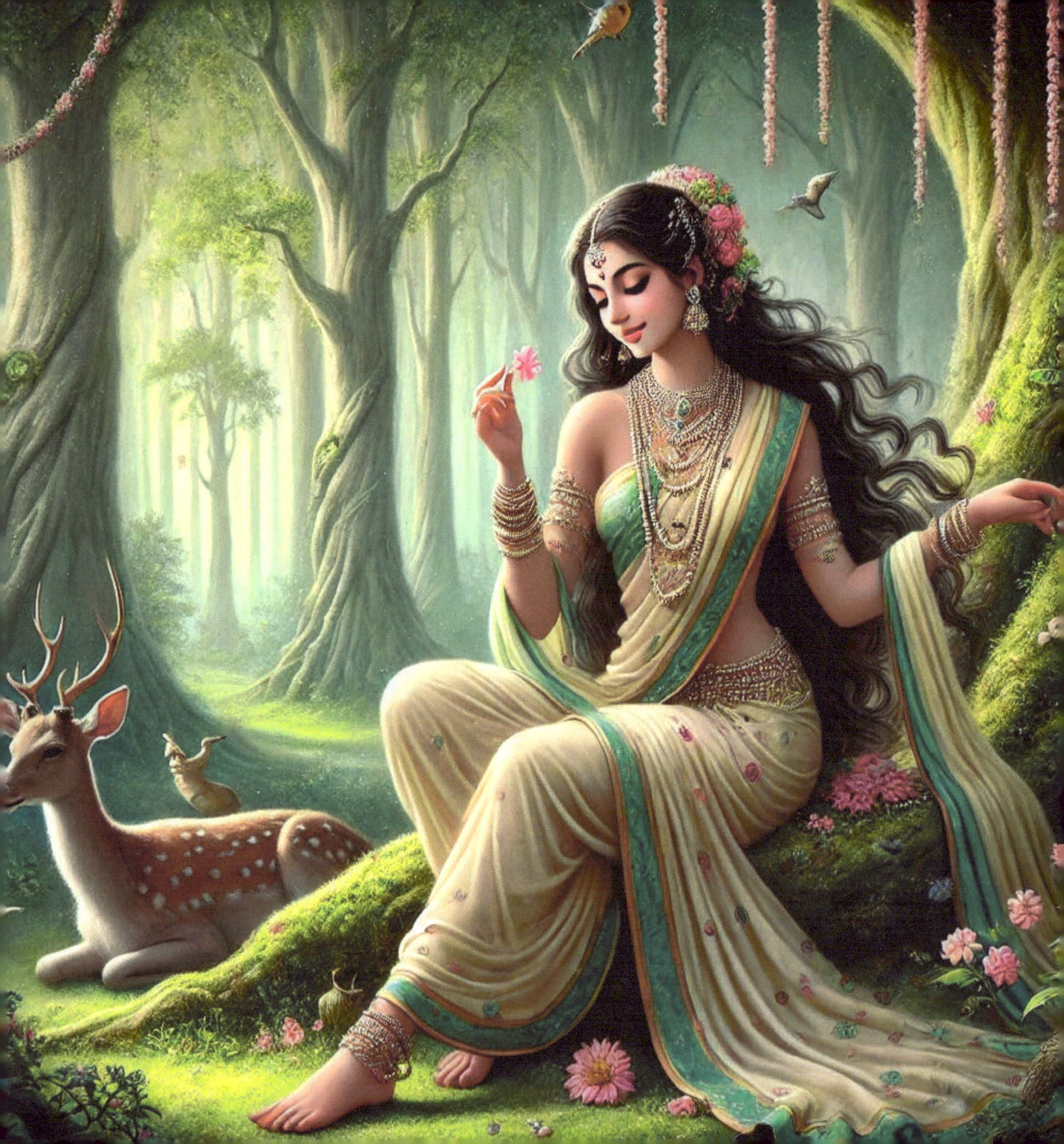

5. From Sorrow to Strength

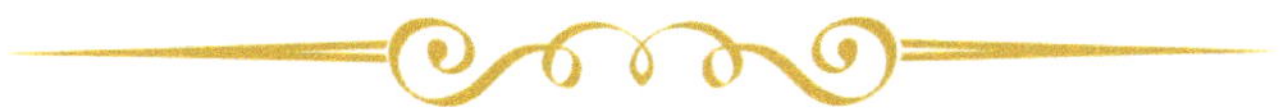

After performing intense penance for thousands of years, Rishi Vishwamitra succumbed to the enchanting beauty of the celestial nymph, Menaka, and their union gave birth to Shakuntala. However, soon after her birth, Vishwamitra, overwhelmed by guilt, left to continue his penance, while Menaka returned to the heavens, leaving the infant Shakuntala behind. She was then adopted by the kind-hearted Rishi Kanva, who raised her with the utmost love and care in his ashram. Under his guidance, Shakuntala blossomed into a woman of extraordinary beauty, inheriting her mother's grace and her father's intelligence.

One day, King Dushyanta of Hastinapura happened to pass by the ashram while on a hunting expedition. Upon seeing Shakuntala, he was instantly captivated by her ethereal beauty, while she, in turn, was charmed by his strength, valour, and royal bearing. They were madly in love with one another and incredibly happy, thus got married secretly. Before departing for his kingdom, King Dushyanta gave Shakuntala his ring as a token of love and commitment promising a royal wedding.

Being left alone, Shakuntala was always engrossed in the joyful recollections of King Dushyanta. One day, when Rishi Durvasa, who was infamous for his nasty temper, visited the ashrama, Shakuntala failed to notice and greet the sage. Furious at the perceived insult, the quick-tempered sage cursed her: "The one in whose thoughts you are lost will forget you entirely unless reminded by a token of love he has given you." Shakuntala, unaware of the curse, continued waiting for Dushyanta and got confused as to why he hadn't returned.

Time passed, and when Shakuntala discovered she was pregnant, she shared her concerns with Rishi Kanva, who decided to take her to King Dushyanta's court. However, upon their arrival at the palace, Dushyanta, under the spell of Durvasa's curse, denied any knowledge of their marriage or her. In desperation, Shakuntala searched for the ring he had given her, only to realise she had lost it during the journey. Heartbroken and humiliated, Shakuntala moved to the forest, devoting herself entirely to the welfare of her unborn child.

In time, Shakuntala gave birth to a son whom she named Bharata. Raised among the wild animals of the forest, Bharata grew to be fearless, courageous, and agile. Shakuntala taught him archery and weaponry and instilled in him the wisdom of the Vedas and Upanishads. Her efforts transformed him into a bold, wise, and righteous person.

Later, when Dushyant came across the ring, he recollected his past and was reunited with his family. Bharata became a legendary brave emperor, the Chakravarti (universal monarch). He played a crucial role in shaping the history of our country, and after his name, the Indian subcontinent was named Bharata.

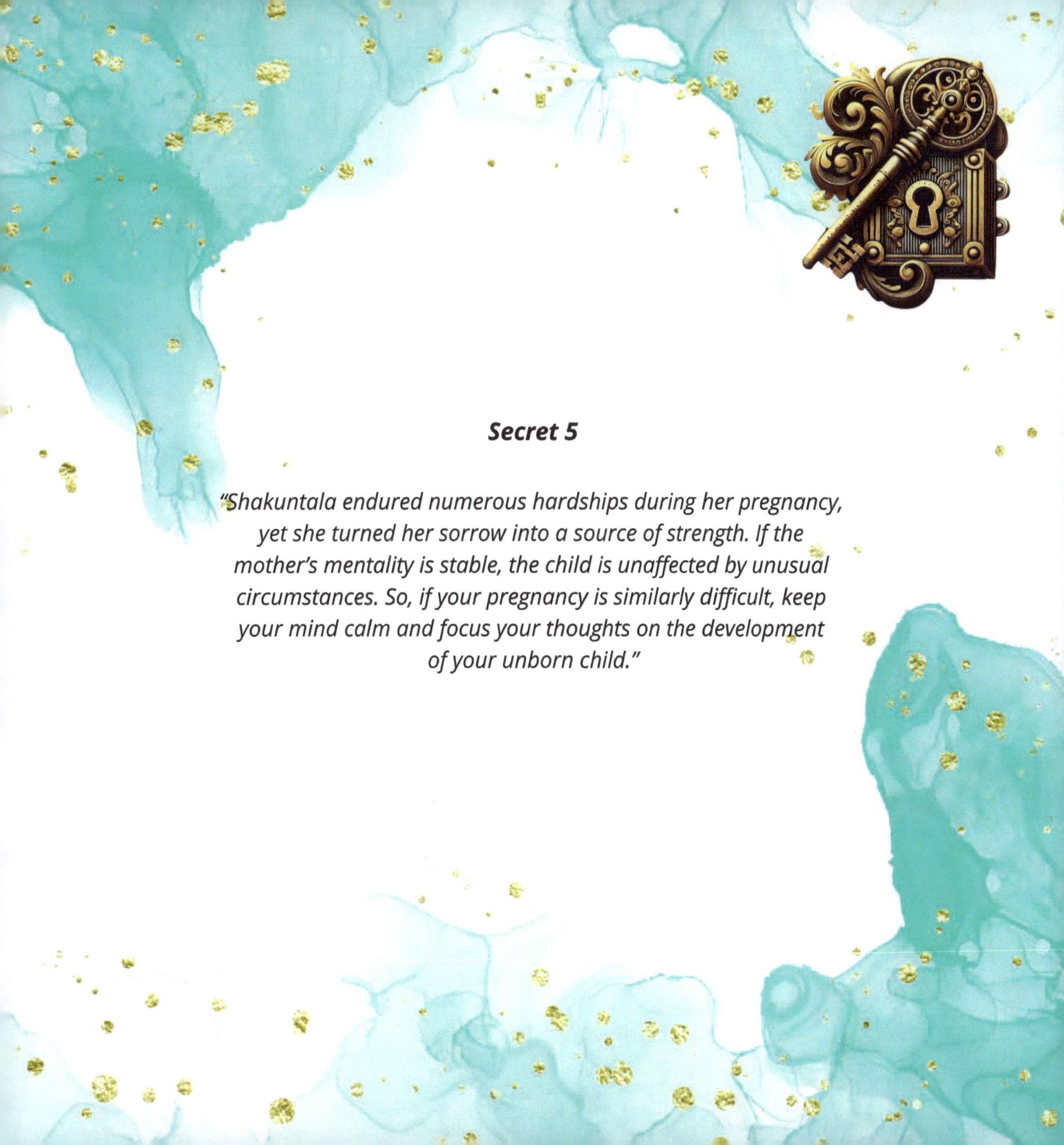

Secret 5

"Shakuntala endured numerous hardships during her pregnancy, yet she turned her sorrow into a source of strength. If the mother's mentality is stable, the child is unaffected by unusual circumstances. So, if your pregnancy is similarly difficult, keep your mind calm and focus your thoughts on the development of your unborn child."

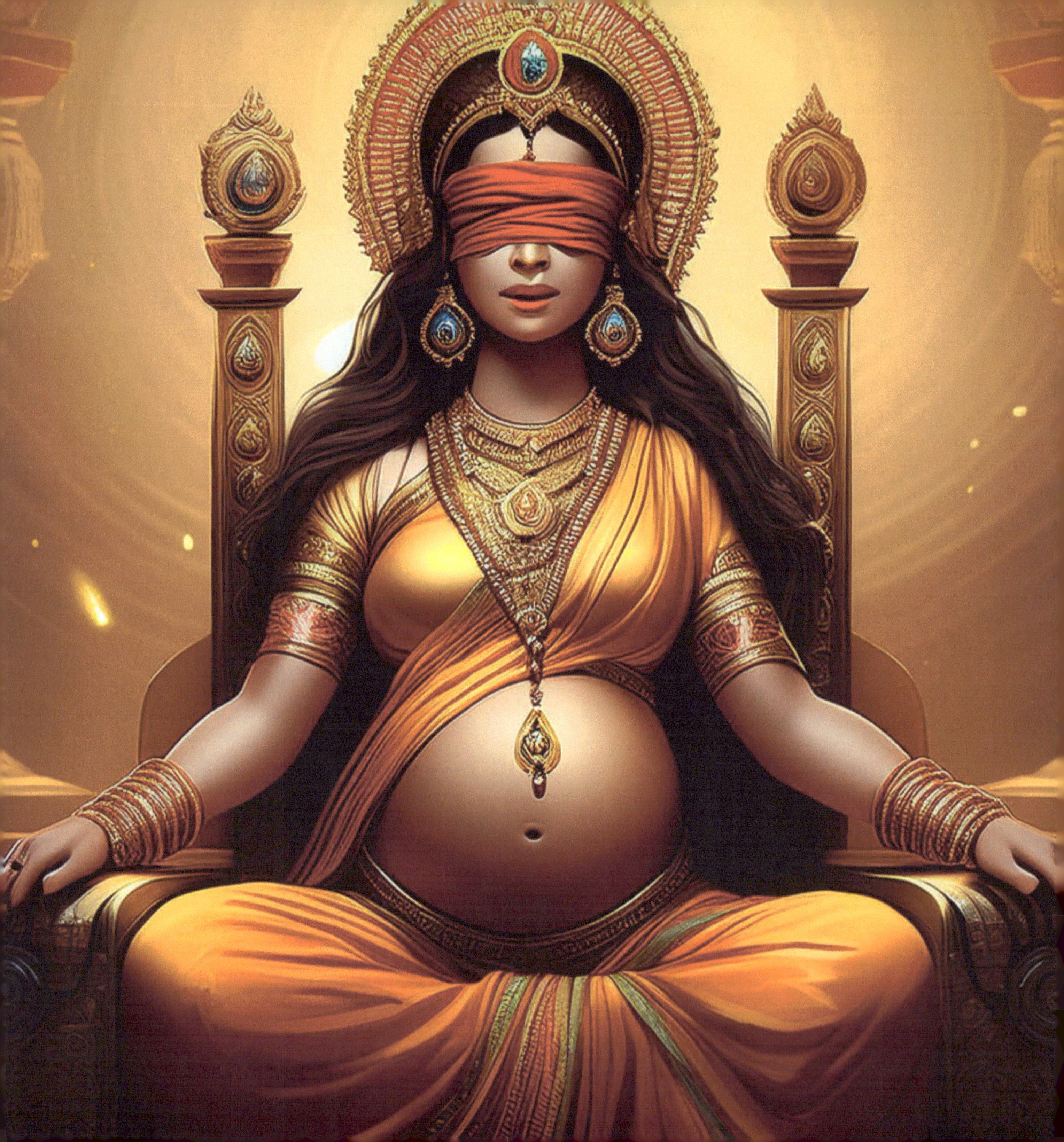

6. Shaping Character

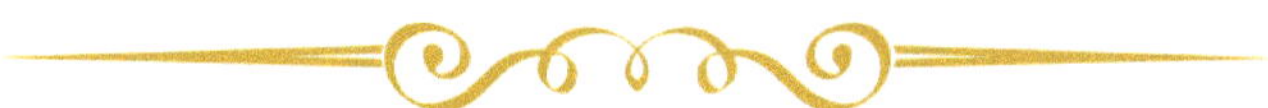

Gandhari was the princess of the ancient Gandhara kingdom, the daughter of King Subala, and the sister of Shakuni. As a mark of her heritage, she was named Gandhari. Known for her extraordinary grace, virtue, and inner strength, she embodied the ideals of a noblewoman, earning widespread respect.

Her marriage was arranged with Dhritarashtra, the eldest prince of the Kuru dynasty. Upon learning that her future husband was born blind, Gandhari made a life-altering decision—to blindfold herself for the rest of her life, choosing to share in Dhritarashtra's darkness. This self-imposed blindness became the ultimate symbol of her sacrifice, love, and unwavering loyalty to her husband.

Despite being the eldest, Dhritarashtra was passed over for the throne due to his blindness. Instead, his younger brother Pandu ascended the throne. However, after a curse by Sage Kindama, Pandu renounced his kingdom to repent in the forests along with his wife Kunti and Madri. Dhritarashtra was crowned king, and Gandhari became queen of Hastinapura.

Gandhari soon became pregnant, but her pregnancy persisted for an exceptionally long time. Meanwhile, Pandu's wife gave birth to a son they called Yudhishthira, followed by Bheema, Arjuna, Nakula, and Sahadeva—the Pandavas. Knowing that the oldest prince would be a strong contender for the throne, Gandhari became envious. Her anxiety and frustration grew as her pregnancy continued without progress. In a moment of desperation,

Gandhari struck her womb, and instead of giving birth to a child, she gave birth to a lump of lifeless flesh.

Distressed and heartbroken, Gandhari turned to the sage Vyasa for help. Vyasa, with his divine power, divided the mass into 101 pieces and placed each piece in a jar filled with milk. After 2 years, the jars were opened, and from them emerged 100 sons and one daughter. The eldest of these sons was Duryodhana, whose birth was marked by ominous signs. Animals howled, winds howled, and unnatural disturbances filled the air, forewarning the coming chaos.

As the Pandavas were very virtuous, courageous, obedient, and full of merit, Duryodhana was immensely jealous of them. Duryodhana saw Yudhishthira as a threat to his ambition of becoming the King of Hastinapura. He, along with his maternal uncle Shakuni, plotted many conspiracies against the Pandavas, including inviting them to the infamous dice game, poisoning Bheema, and setting them on fire in Lakshya Graha. His intense animosity and jealousy sparked the Mahabharata war, in which the Kauravas sadly perished. In just 18 days, 1,660 million warriors lost their lives in the Kurukshetra War, and only 12 major warriors survived the war. Duryodhana's greed and arrogance led to his downfall in the Mahabharata."

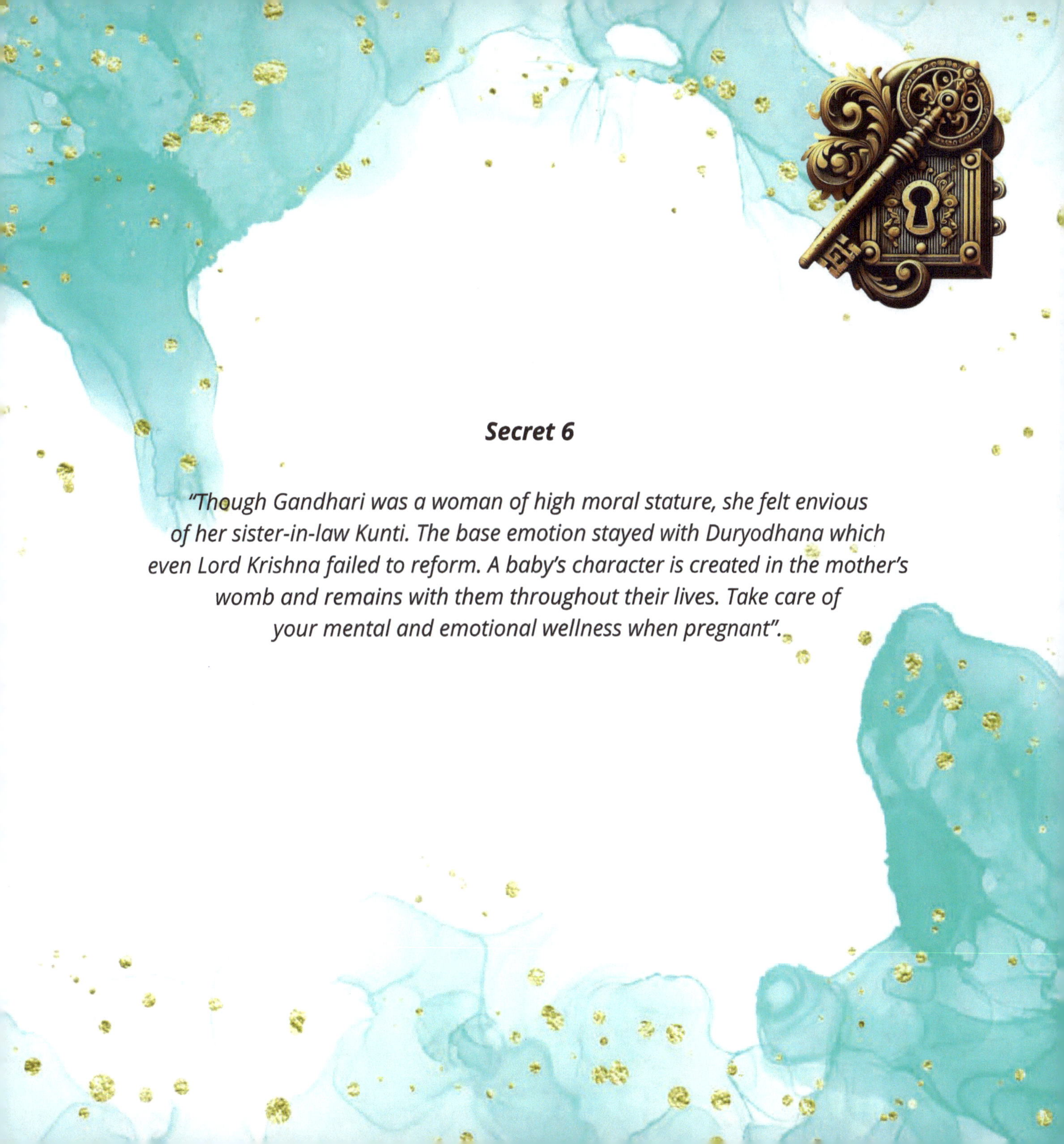

Secret 6

"Though Gandhari was a woman of high moral stature, she felt envious of her sister-in-law Kunti. The base emotion stayed with Duryodhana which even Lord Krishna failed to reform. A baby's character is created in the mother's womb and remains with them throughout their lives. Take care of your mental and emotional wellness when pregnant".

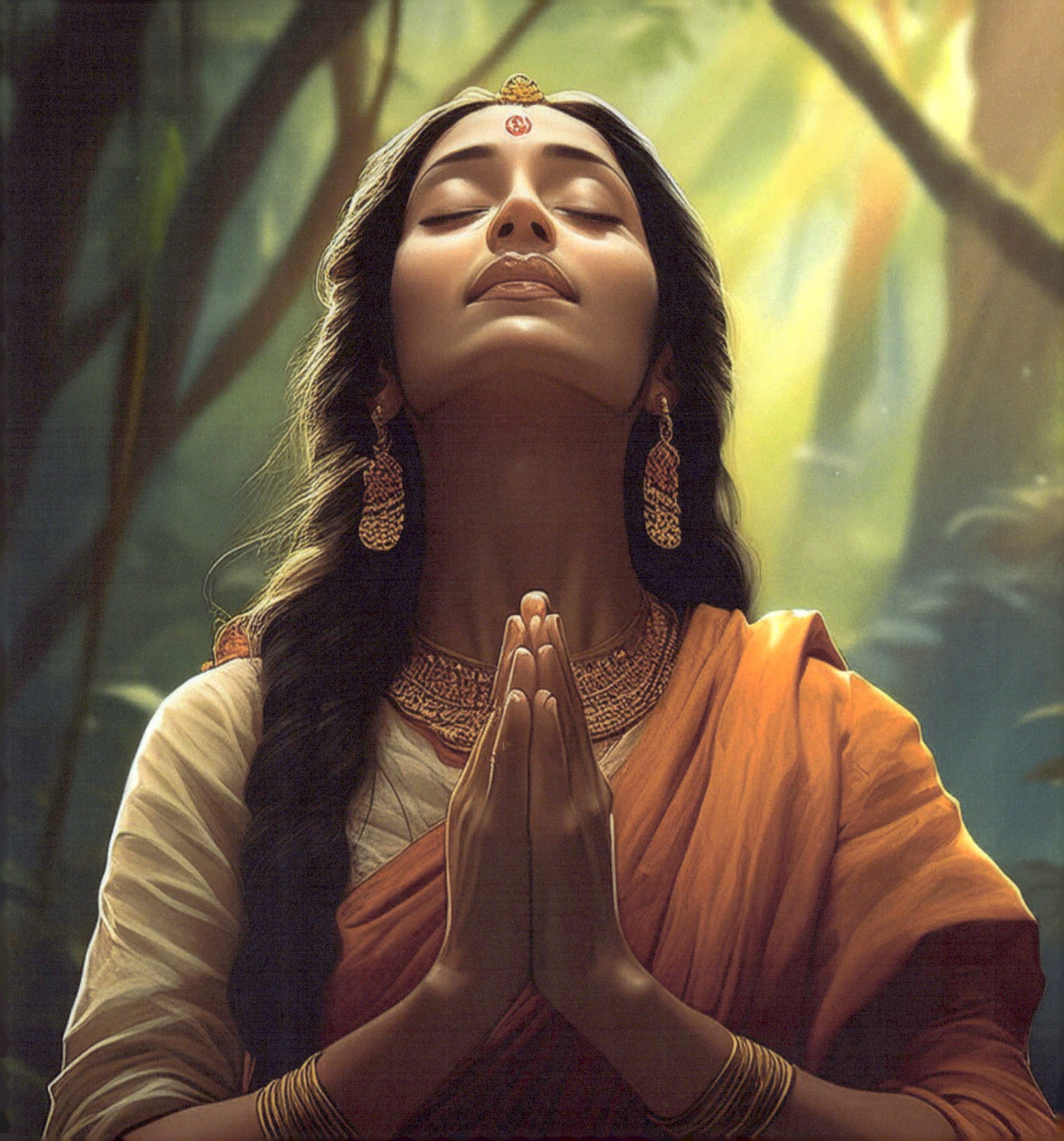

7. Fruits of Karma

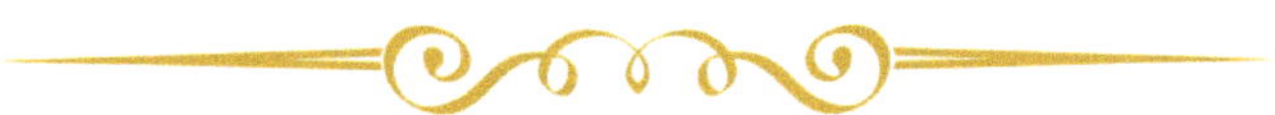

Kunti was a daughter of Surasena from the Yadu clan and was initially named Pritha. She was thus the sister of Vasudeva, father of Krishna. Later, she was adopted by King Kuntibhoja, her father's cousin, as he was childless and was renamed Kunti. After her arrival, King Kuntibhoja was blessed with children, which was why King Kuntibhoja considered her his fortunate charm and took excellent care of her. She grew into a beautiful, intelligent, and wise princess, admired by all.

One day, the famous sage Durvasa, notorious for his short temper and powerful curses, visited King Kuntibhoja's kingdom. Kunti, young but dutiful, was tasked with serving him during his stay. Her patience and dedication greatly pleased the sage, who blessed her with a unique boon – a secret chant that would allow her to summon any god and have a child with them without the need for pregnancy.

When Kunti reached the age of marriage, King Surasena arranged a grand swayamvara for her. Princes from far and wide attended, but it was Pandu, a skilled archer and warrior, who won her hand. Soon after, Pandu also married Madri, the princess of the Madra Kingdom. Under Pandu's leadership, the Kuru empire expanded greatly, as he conquered numerous kingdoms including Sindhu, Kashi, Anga, Trigarta, Kalinga, and Magadha.

However, Pandu's life took a tragic turn when, while hunting, he accidentally shot the Sage Kindama and his wife, mistaking them for deer in the forest. In his dying moments, Kindama cursed Pandu, declaring that he would die if he ever tried to be intimate with his wives. That means he must stay childless to stay alive. Filled with remorse, grief-stricken Pandu abandoned his kingdom and fled to the jungle with his wife to perform penance.

Seeing Pandu's anguish, Kunti revealed the secret mantra bestowed upon her by sage Durvasa. With his consent, she invoked the gods to grant them children. First, she called upon Yama, the God of Dharma, who blessed her with Yudhishthira. Then, she summoned Vayu, the wind god, and gave birth to Bhima. Finally, she invoked Indra, the king of gods, and bore Arjuna. Out of compassion for her co-wife, Kunti shared the mantra with Madri, who used it to summon the Ashvins, twin gods, resulting in the birth of Nakula and Sahadeva.

These 5 brothers, known as the Pandavas, grew up to be central figures in the Mahabharata. Their rivalry with their cousins, the Kauravas, over the throne of Hastinapur culminated in the great Kurukshetra War, where the Pandavas ultimately triumphed, establishing Dharma.

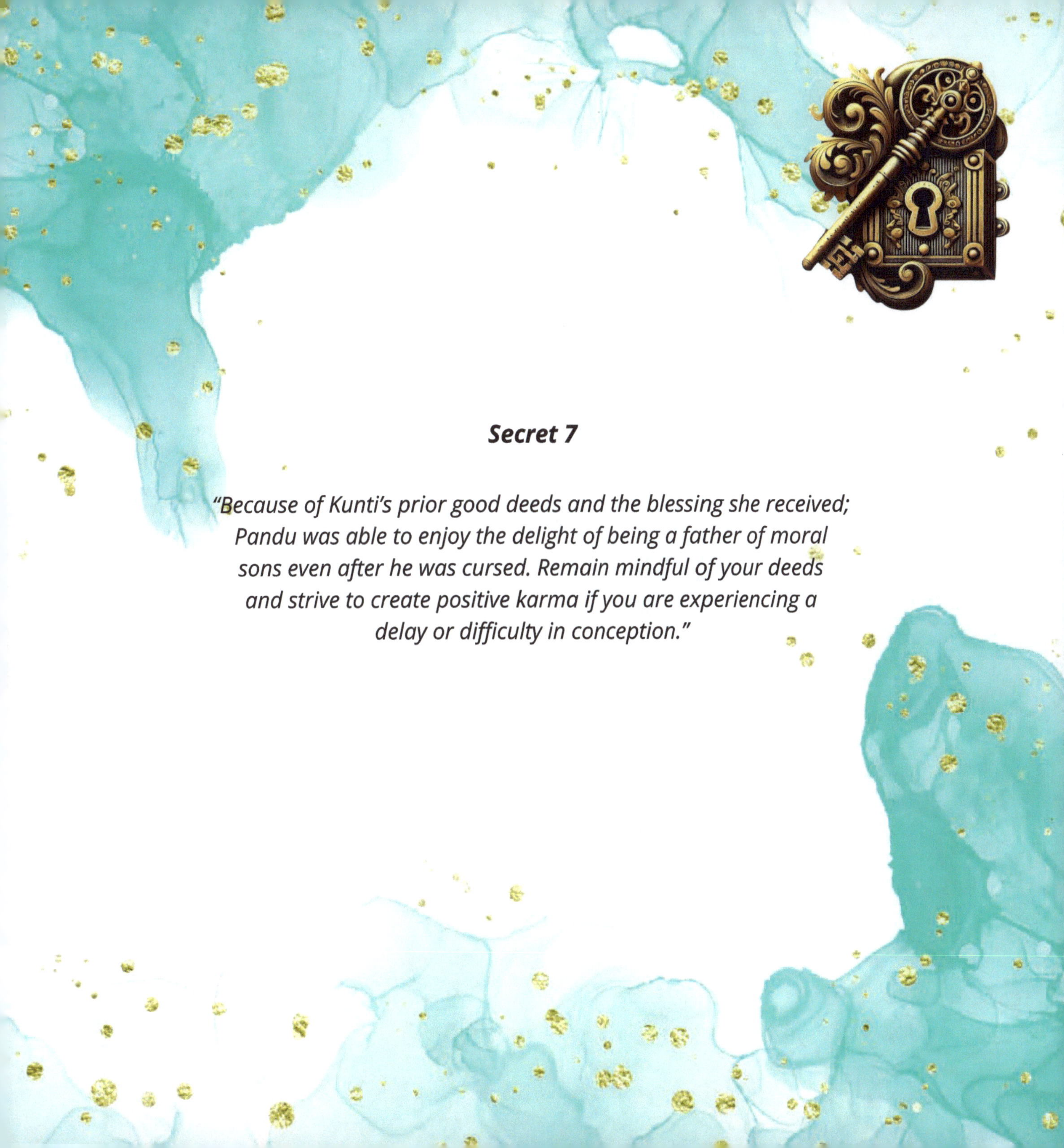

Secret 7

"Because of Kunti's prior good deeds and the blessing she received; Pandu was able to enjoy the delight of being a father of moral sons even after he was cursed. Remain mindful of your deeds and strive to create positive karma if you are experiencing a delay or difficulty in conception."

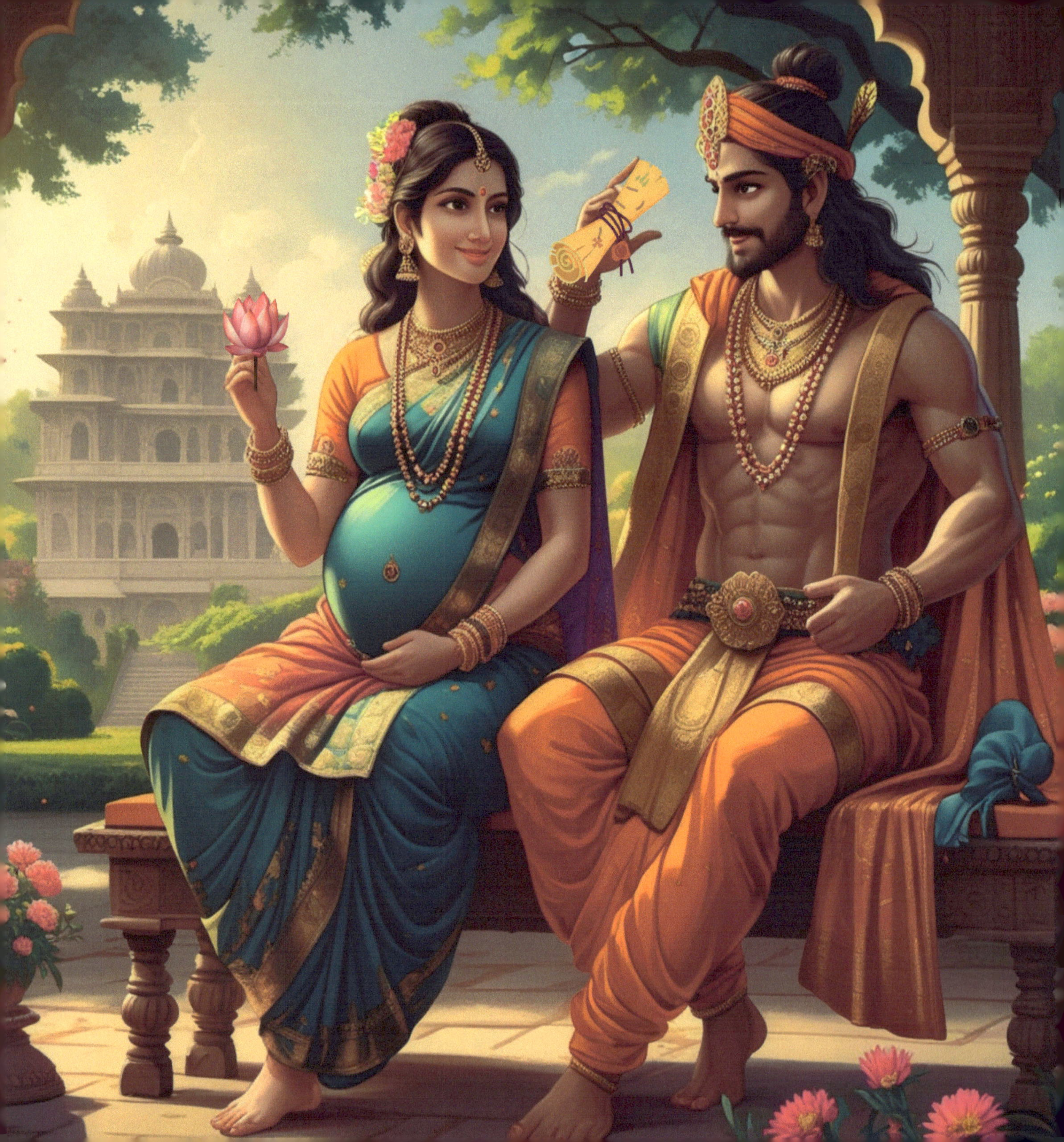

8. Womb: The First School

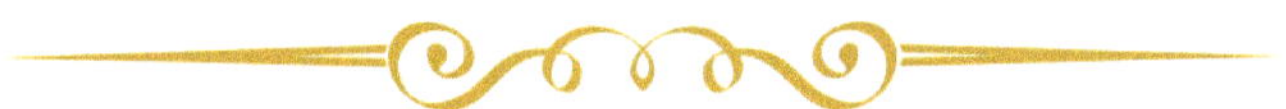

Subhadra was the daughter of Vasudeva and Rohini Devi and a beloved half-sister of Lord Krishna. She was born after Krishna rescued his father, Vasudeva, from imprisonment, and as a result, she enjoyed the comforts of royalty, escaping the pain that had haunted her family before her birth. Devi Subhadra was trained in disciplines like Statecraft, Politics, and Diplomacy. Being a warrior, Subhadra was proficient with all types of weaponry. She was the world's finest charioteer as she was personally trained by Krishna.

As fate would have it, during Arjuna's exile—a consequence of breaking his vow—he sought refuge in Dwaraka, where he lived with his cousin Krishna. It was here that he fell deeply in love with Subhadra, who, in turn, was equally captivated by his valour and charm. Their love blossomed, culminating in a marriage, a union forged in shared interests and mutual respect.

Subhadra was so fascinated by warfare and different formations that she once asked Arjuna about the chakravyuha formation. Arjuna was narrating the strategy of entering the chakravyuha with no awareness that the baby Abhimanyu in the womb was very attentively listening to this conversation and was grasping the very secretive knowledge of advancing through the chakravyuha. Arjuna halted the tale because Subhadra dozed off in between. Unfortunately, Abhimanyu gained only half the knowledge and did not know how to emerge from the chakravyuha successfully.

After the Pandavas left for exile following the ill-fated dice game, Krishna took on the responsibility of raising Abhimanyu, who was only 2 years old at the time. Pradyumna, Krishna's son, became his teacher and provided excellent training. Perfect guidance and humble nature, coupled with a great inheritance, made Abhimanyu the most heroic and skilled.

On the 13th day of the epic Mahabharata war, Guru Drona, commander-in-chief of the Kauravas, devised the chakravyuha that only a handful knew how to shatter. Only Krishna and Arjuna in the Pandavas' camp knew this knowledge. Guru Drona kept Arjuna and Krishna busy with the Samsaptakhas army away from the battlefield. Abhimanyu came to the Pandavas' rescue and entered the battle formation all alone, despite just knowing how to enter it.

So great was his valour that even eminent warriors could not stand against this 16-year-old boy. When they couldn't overcome him, they turned to treachery. Guru Drona, Karna, Shakuni, Duryodhana, Kritvarma, and Shalya all attacked him at the same time and killed him in the most gruesome manner. There was not a single part of his body where he was not wounded. In many ways, Abhimanyu's death marked a turning point in the Mahabharata conflict. It altered the Pandavas' mentality, making reconciliation impossible.

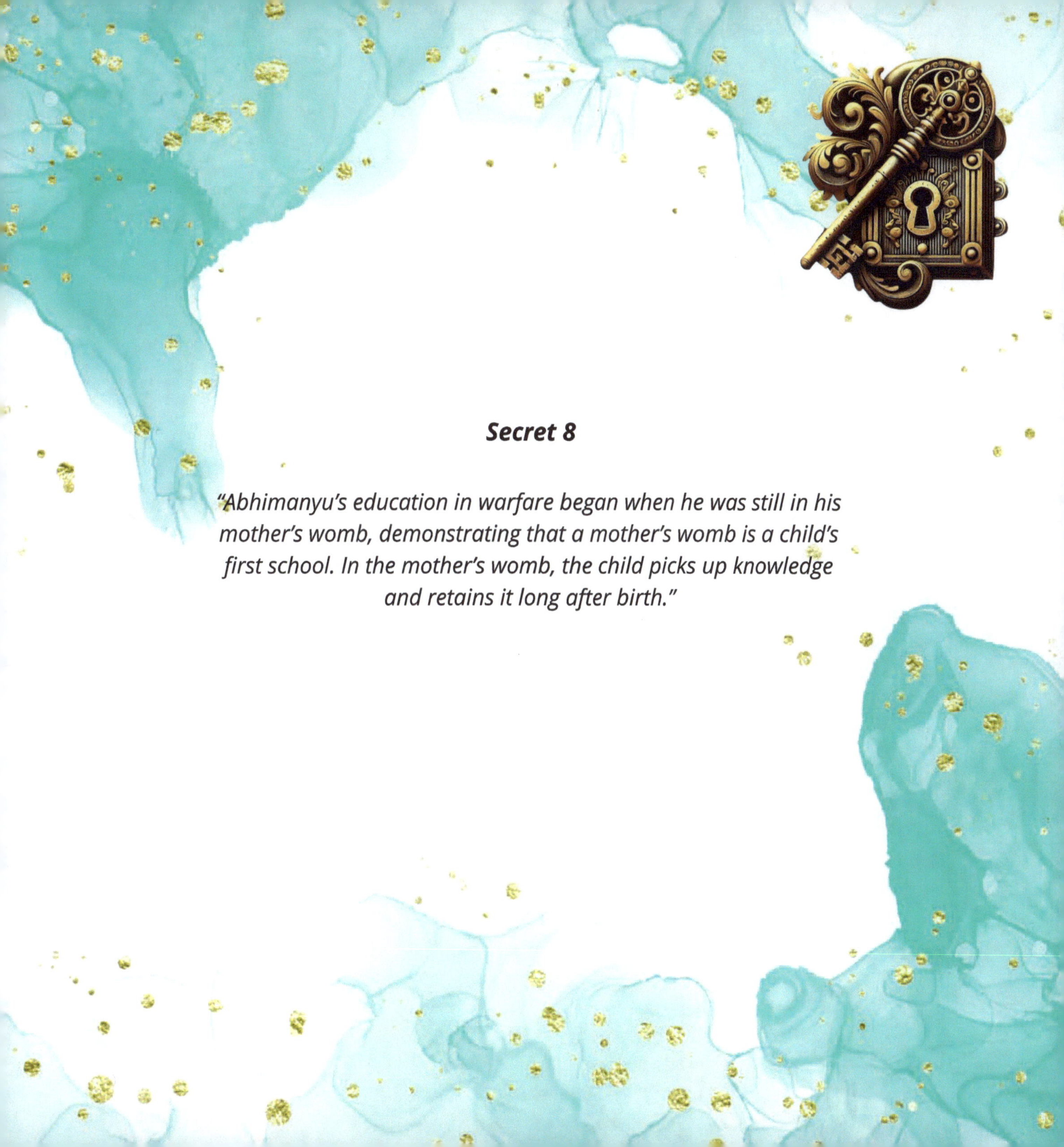

Secret 8

"Abhimanyu's education in warfare began when he was still in his mother's womb, demonstrating that a mother's womb is a child's first school. In the mother's womb, the child picks up knowledge and retains it long after birth."

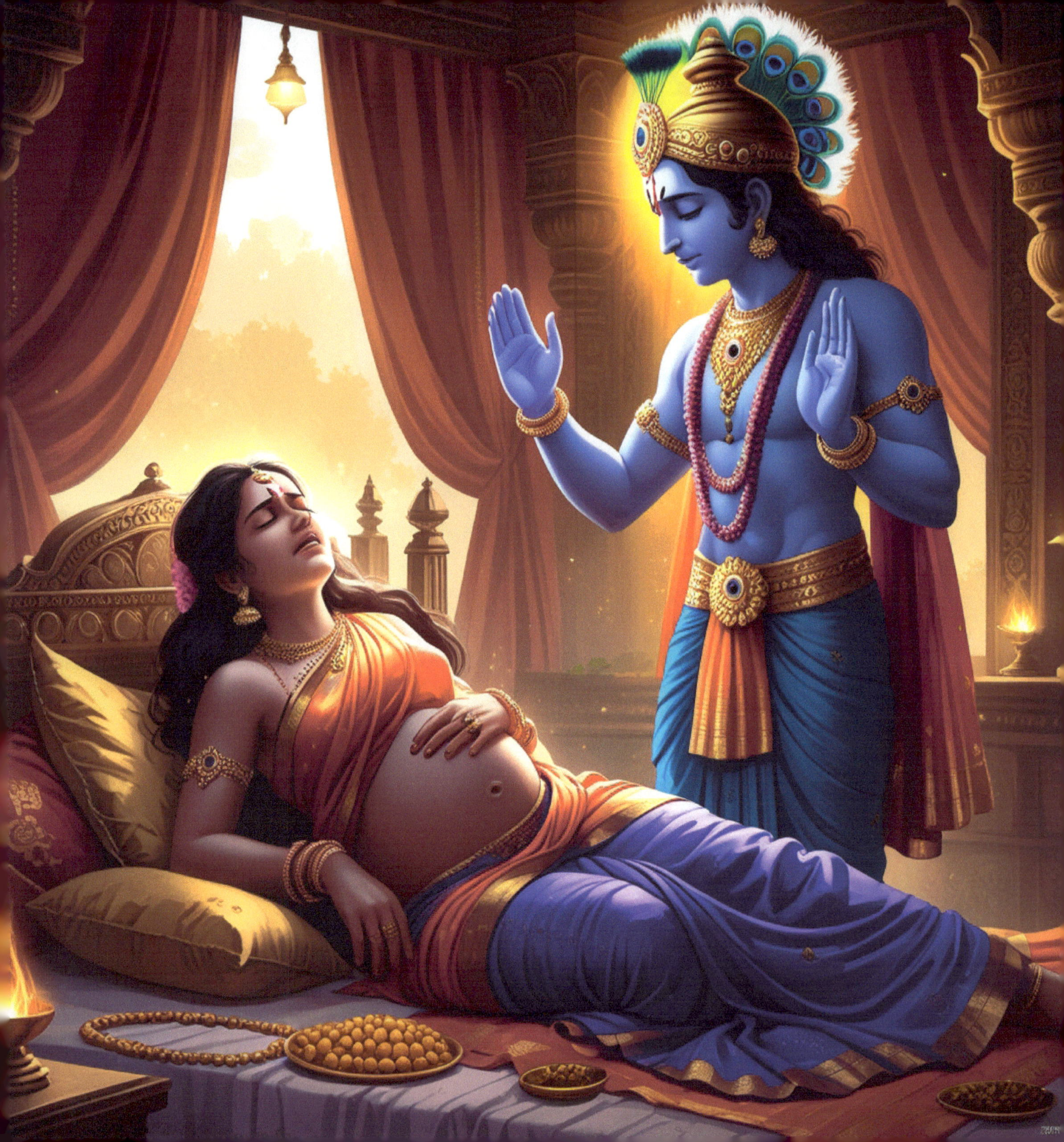

9. Prenatal Consciousness

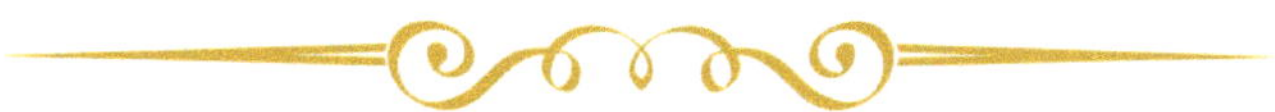

Uttara was the beloved daughter of King Virata, the ruler of the Matsya kingdom. Known for her piety and grace, she was married to Abhimanyu, the son of Arjuna and Subhadra. Their union was a joyful one, but fate took a cruel turn when Abhimanyu was killed mercilessly by the Kauravas while Uttara was in the advanced stages of pregnancy. The sight of her husband's lifeless body shattered her heart, leaving her widowed at such a young age, at a moment when she needed him the most. Overwhelmed by grief, she found solace in the comforting presence of Lord Krishna.

At the end of the Kurukshetra War, most of the warriors had perished. From the Pandava camp, few remained, and from the Kauravas' side, only 4 were alive: Duryodhana, Kripacharya, Kritavarman, and Ashwatthama. Bhim, the Pandava, had defeated Duryodhana and was badly wounded. Driven by fury, Ashwatthama infiltrated the Pandava camp with the intent to kill them. In his blind rage, he brutally murdered the sleeping sons of the Pandavas, mistaking them for their fathers.

The next morning, Draupadi's heart was torn apart by the devastating news of her sons' deaths. The Pandavas were horrified and plunged into despair. Arjuna went after Ashwatthama to take revenge while Krishna also followed. Sensing the rage in Arjuna's eyes, Ashwatthama was filled with fear. Realising he could not triumph through conventional means, he invoked the Brahmastra, a weapon of immense power. When Arjuna fired a Brahmastra to match, Narada and Vyasa intervened, commanding both men to withdraw their weapons. While Arjuna complied, Ashwatthama, still consumed by anger, redirected his Brahmastra towards Uttara's womb, intending to obliterate the unborn child and extinguish the Pandava lineage.

Uttara cried out for help, and in response to her desperate plea, Lord Krishna, in his divine grace, entered her womb in a subtle form. Brahmastra had already impacted and killed the baby in the womb. Lord Krishna pacified the Brahmastra and enlivened the womb again. He gave Darshan to the unborn child in the womb.

When the child was eventually born, he exhibited unusual behaviour by constantly looking around as if searching for something. The youngster was searching everywhere for Lord Krishna after having a magnificent vision of the Lord while still in the womb. As a result, he was named Parikshita, meaning "looking around intently."

As Parikshit grew, he would inherit the throne of Hastinapur, becoming a renowned ruler known for establishing a just and dharmic kingdom. His reign was marked by fairness and righteousness, a legacy that honoured the sacrifices of his parents and the guiding light of Lord Krishna.

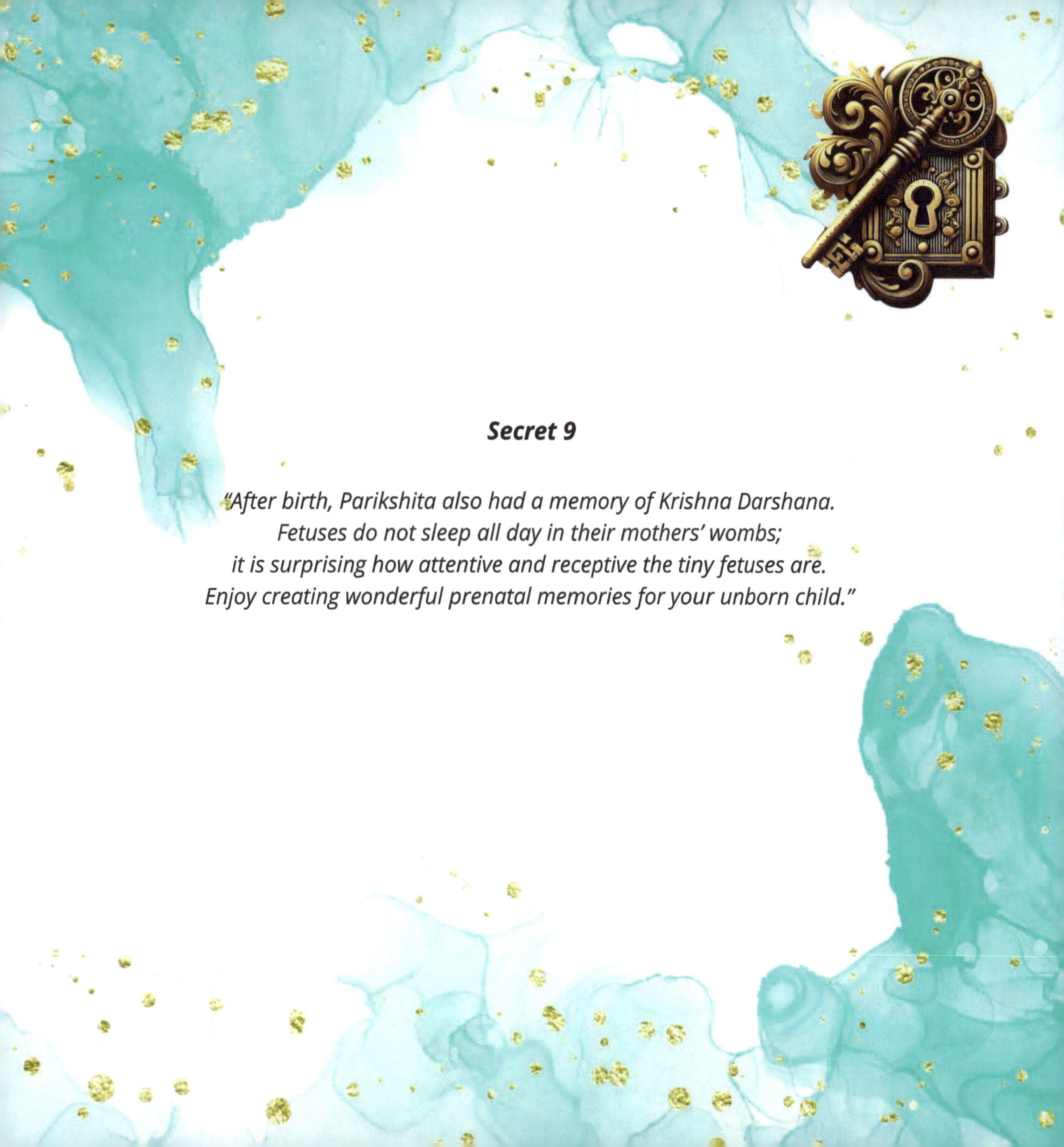

Secret 9

*"After birth, Parikshita also had a memory of Krishna Darshana.
Fetuses do not sleep all day in their mothers' wombs;
it is surprising how attentive and receptive the tiny fetuses are.
Enjoy creating wonderful prenatal memories for your unborn child."*

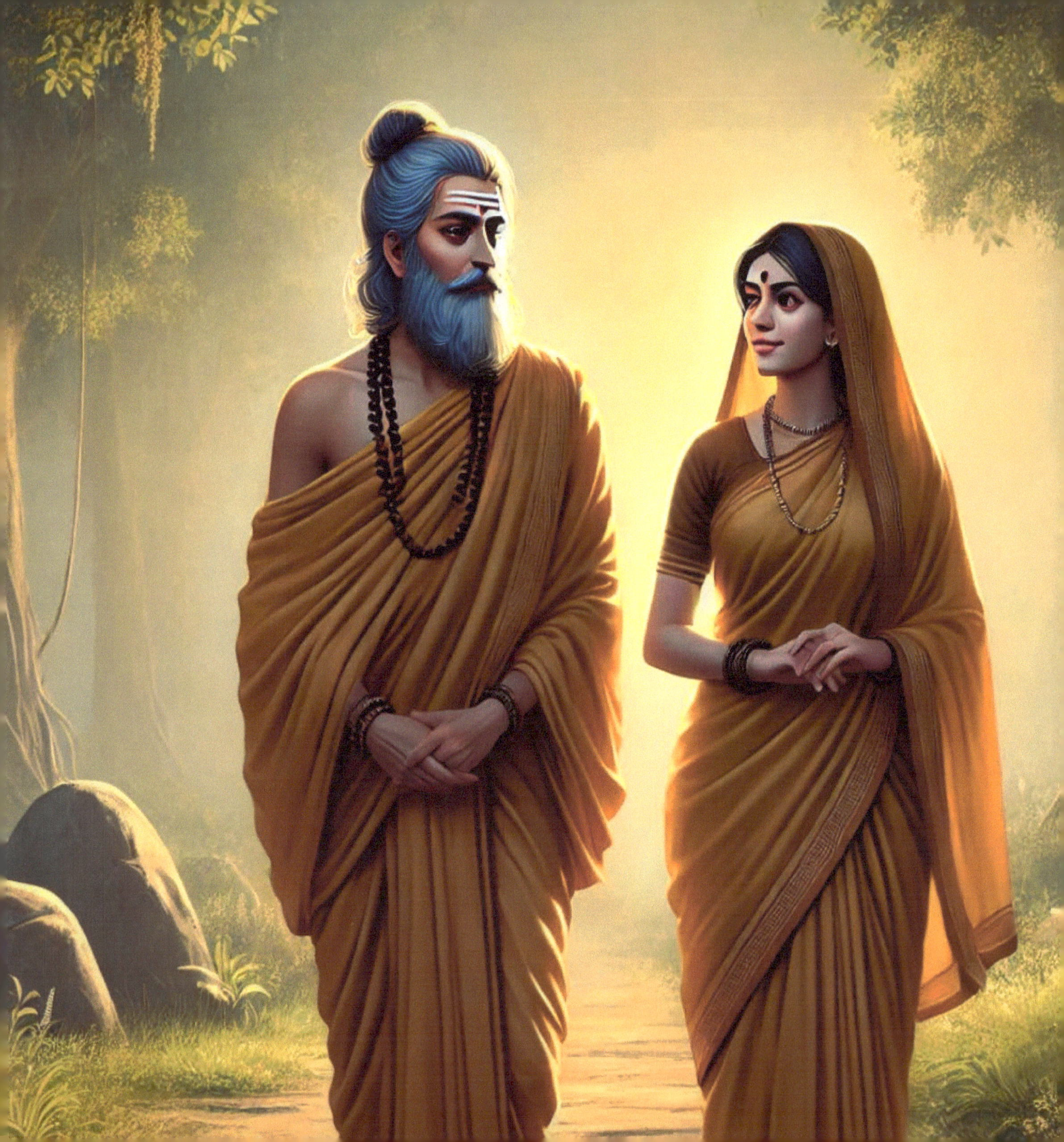

10. Seeds of Devotion

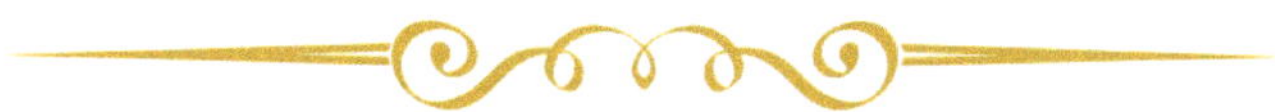

Mrikandu was the son of Sage Bringu and, like his father, he was a revered sage. He was married to the noblewoman Marudvati. The couple was leading a happy married life but for a long time, they didn't bear any children. Both were ardent devotees of Lord Shiva, so they started praying to him. Delighted with their devotion, Lord Shiva appeared before Mrikandu and posed a profound choice: "Would you prefer a hundred sons who will lead long, foolish lives or a single wise son who will only live for 16 years?" After a moment of contemplation, Mrikandu replied, "O Lord, please bless me with that one wise son." "Tathastu," Lord Shiva granted his wish.

Soon after, Marudvati became pregnant and gave birth to a son named Markandeya. Markandeya was exceptionally intelligent, wise, and handsome, grasping the teachings of the Vedas and Shastras effortlessly. Observing his parents, Markandeya also became a devout follower of Lord Shiva.

Mrikandu Rishi started growing sad as Markandeya was reaching 16. Unable to understand his father's misery, Markandeya enquired, "Father, why do you look so low these days?" With a heavy heart, Rishi narrated the entire story to his son and said, "Son, how will we bear the pain of losing you? We will be completely shattered."

Markandeya comforted his father, assuring him that Lord Shiva had always protected his devotees as his own children. Determined to show his devotion, Markandeya built a

Shiva Lingam by the seashore and began to worship Lord Shiva with fervour, reciting the mantra "Om Namah Shivaya," singing bhajans and dancing with joy.

As Markandeya's sixteenth birthday arrived, Yama, the God of Death, appeared before him, stating, "Your time on earth has come. Please come with me." At that moment, Markandeya clung to the Shiva Lingam, refusing to leave. In a fit of anger, Yama attempted to pull him away, but the force of his actions caused the Shiva Lingam to burst open, revealing Lord Shiva in all his glory. Shiva commanded Yama to let Markendeya go, and Yama, compelled to obey, could do nothing but comply. From that day forward, Shiva was known as Kalantaka, the "Ender of Death."

When Markandeya returned home, his parents were overjoyed and expressed their heartfelt gratitude to Lord Shiva for sparing their son's life.

Markandeya grew to be a great sage, authoring the "Markandeya Purana," which contains 137 chapters exploring themes of Dharma, karma, Samsara, and Śrāddha. The Purana comprises 9,000 verses covering a vast array of subjects, including mythology, religion, and societal issues. As one of the Chiranjeevis, immortal beings, Markandeya's story stands as a testament to the power of faith and perseverance, inspiring countless individuals even to this day.

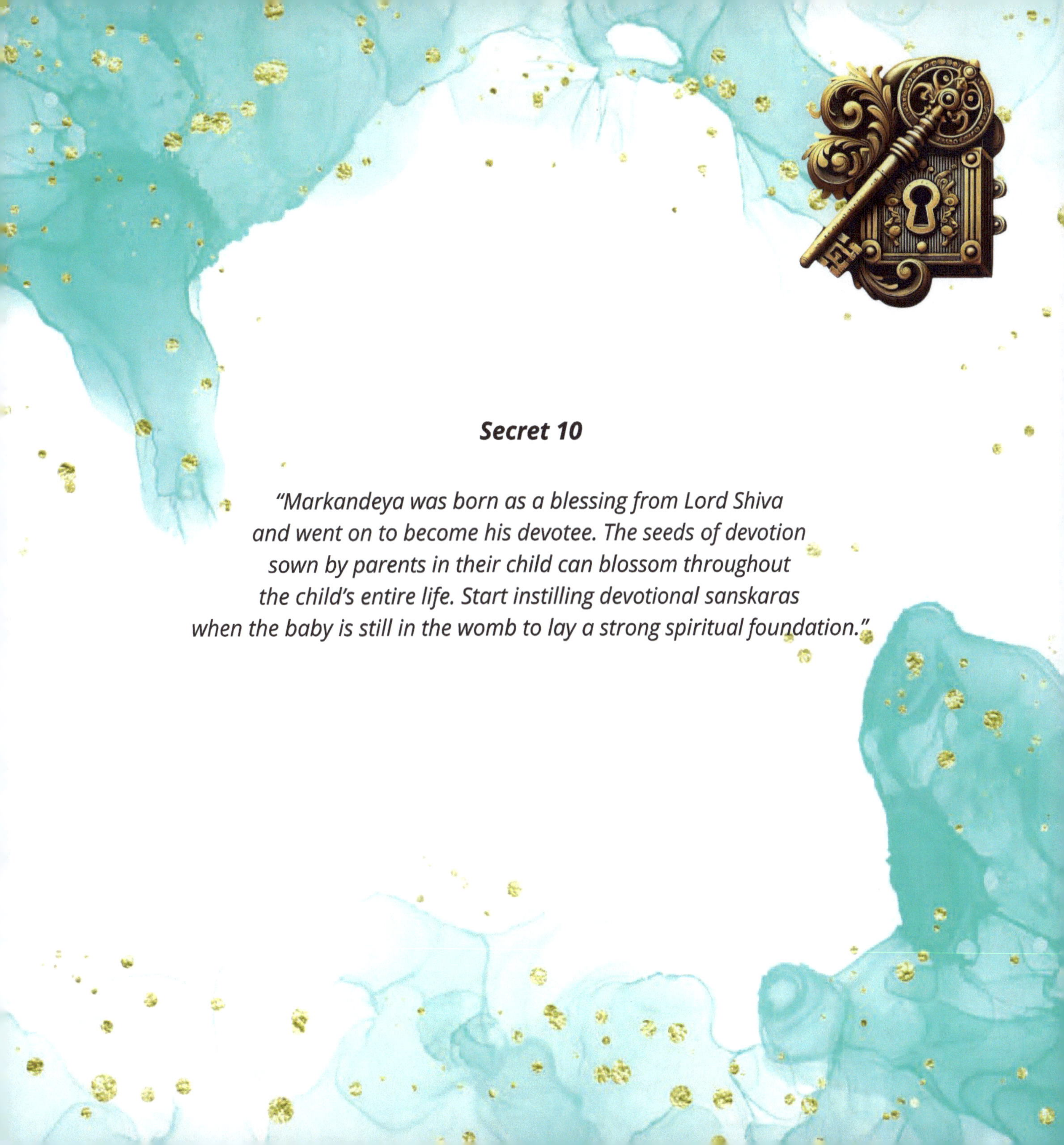

Secret 10

*"Markandeya was born as a blessing from Lord Shiva
and went on to become his devotee. The seeds of devotion
sown by parents in their child can blossom throughout
the child's entire life. Start instilling devotional sanskaras
when the baby is still in the womb to lay a strong spiritual foundation."*

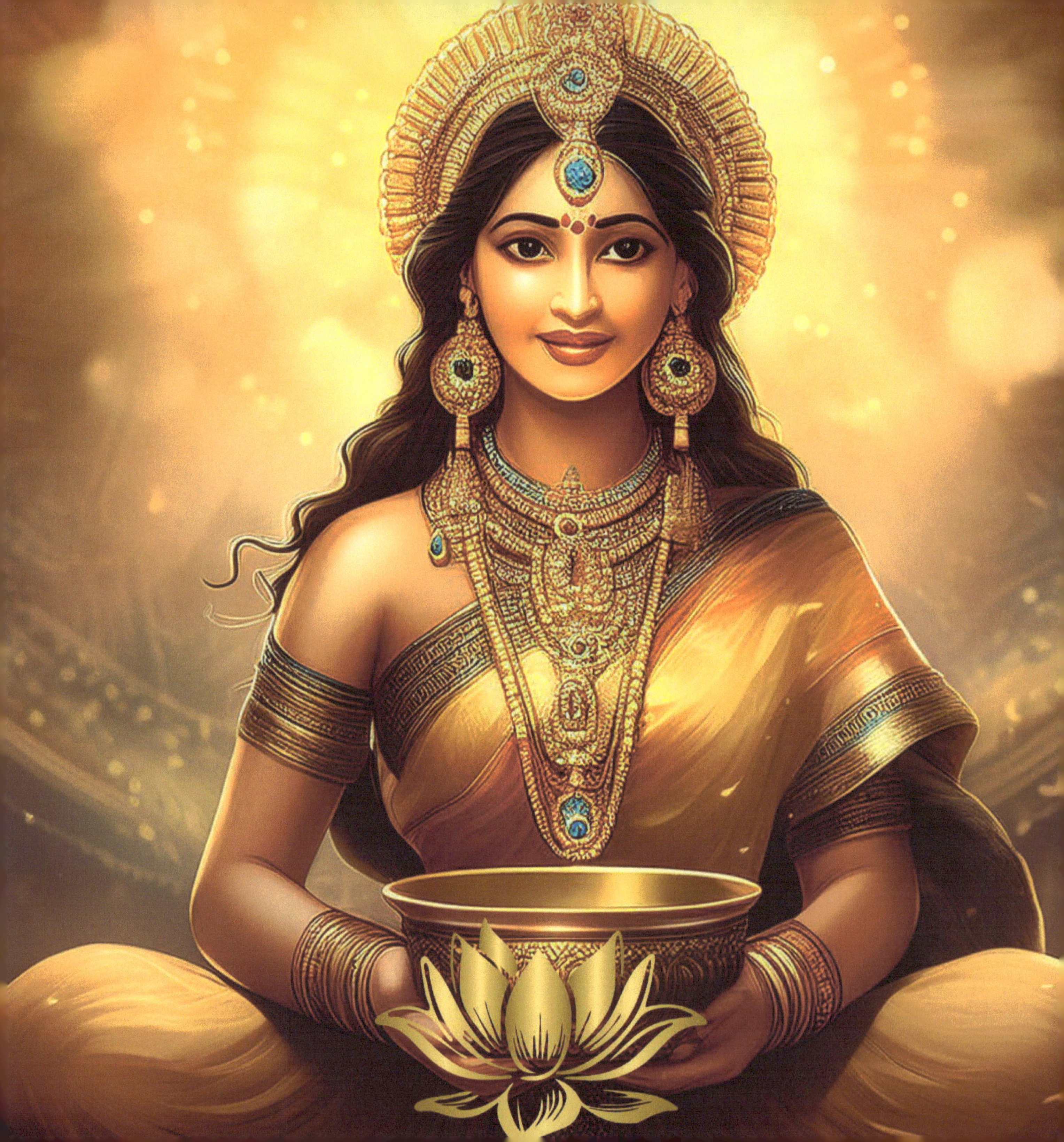

11. Act of Purification

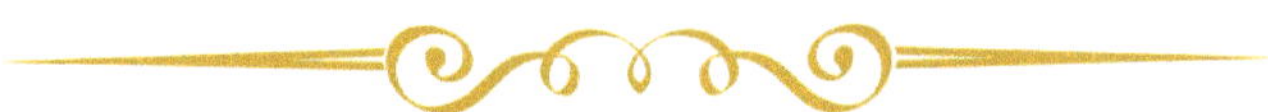

In the ancient kingdom of Uttar Kosala, where fertile fields met blue skies, there lived a graceful princess named Kausalya. Her skillfulness, beauty, and wisdom shone brightly, captivating all who knew her. Eventually, she wed Dasharatha, the mighty king ruling from the majestic city of Ayodhya in Dakshin Kosala. Dasharatha, known as the "King of the Law," was revered for his unwavering commitment to justice and virtue. Despite being Dasharatha's chief wife, she was compassionate and humble. Even when Dasharatha later got married to Sumitra and Kaikeyi, Kausalya treated them like her own sisters and loved them dearly.

Years passed, but no child was born to Dasharatha. He performed many austerities to have a son, but all the efforts were futile, and the throne remained without an heir. Witnessing the King's agony, the royal priest Sage Vasishta suggested seeking the help of sage Rishyasringa. With hope glimmering in his heart, Dasharatha approached Rishyasringa, who recommended performing the sacred Putrakameshti Yagna – an offering to the divine for the boon of children.

A remarkable arrangement was established by King Dasharatha to ensure the triumph of Yagna. He invited all the learned Brahmins and all the priests who were well-versed in Vedas. Vamadeva, Jabali, Kashyapa, and the royal priest Vasistha also joined the ceremony. Rishi Rishyasringa along with Brahmins and sages chanted the Putrakameshti Yagna's prescribed sacred mantras.

Finally, as the flames danced in Yagna's hearth, a divine being emerged from the fire, bearing a celestial offering of kheer—a sweet, milky delicacy. "Share this with Kausalya, Sumitra, and Kaikeyi," the divine figure instructed. Each queen received a portion, and soon after, they were blessed with the joy of pregnancy.

Kaushalya experienced happiness, tranquillity, and calmness when she was pregnant. She often used to feel like slaying the demons. After some time, Kaushalya gave birth to Rama, Sumitra to Lakshmana, and Shatrughna, Kaikeyi to Bharata – the 4 princes were virtuous, brave, and noble.

However, the joy was short-lived. Dasharatha had decided to crown Rama as his heir, but on the eve of the grand ceremony, Kaikeyi, driven by jealousy and ambition, demanded that Dasharatha banish Rama to the forest for 14 years and instead install Bharata as king. "You must honour your promise to me, my lord!" she insisted, her eyes gleaming with determination. Rama went into exile with his wife Seeta and brother Lakshman. Kausalya was inconsolable, but soon she gathered her composure and forgave the king when he sought forgiveness. She did not even blame Kaikeyi for her unfair acts as she was a believer in Karma.

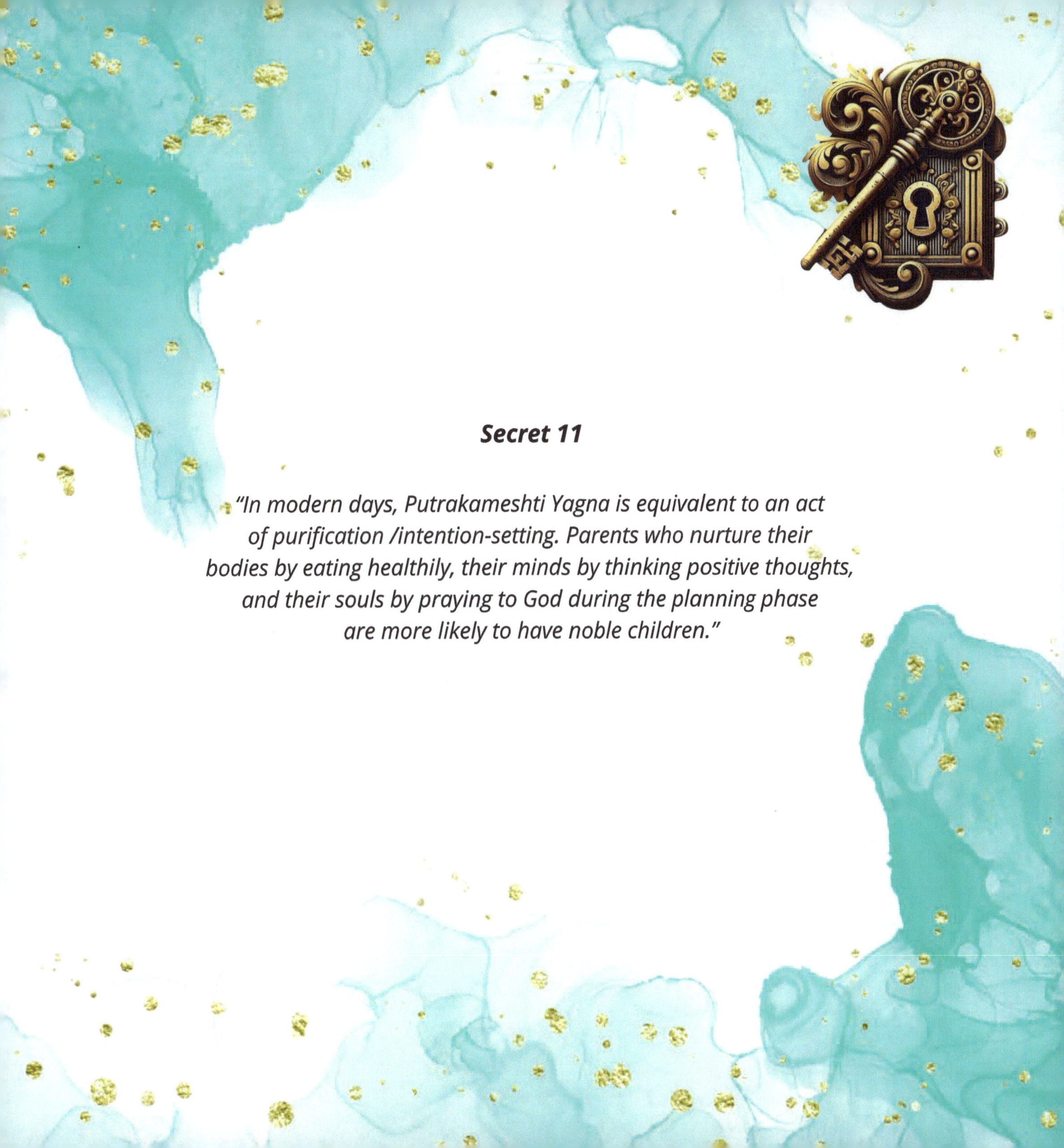

Secret 11

*"In modern days, Putrakameshti Yagna is equivalent to an act
of purification /intention-setting. Parents who nurture their
bodies by eating healthily, their minds by thinking positive thoughts,
and their souls by praying to God during the planning phase
are more likely to have noble children."*

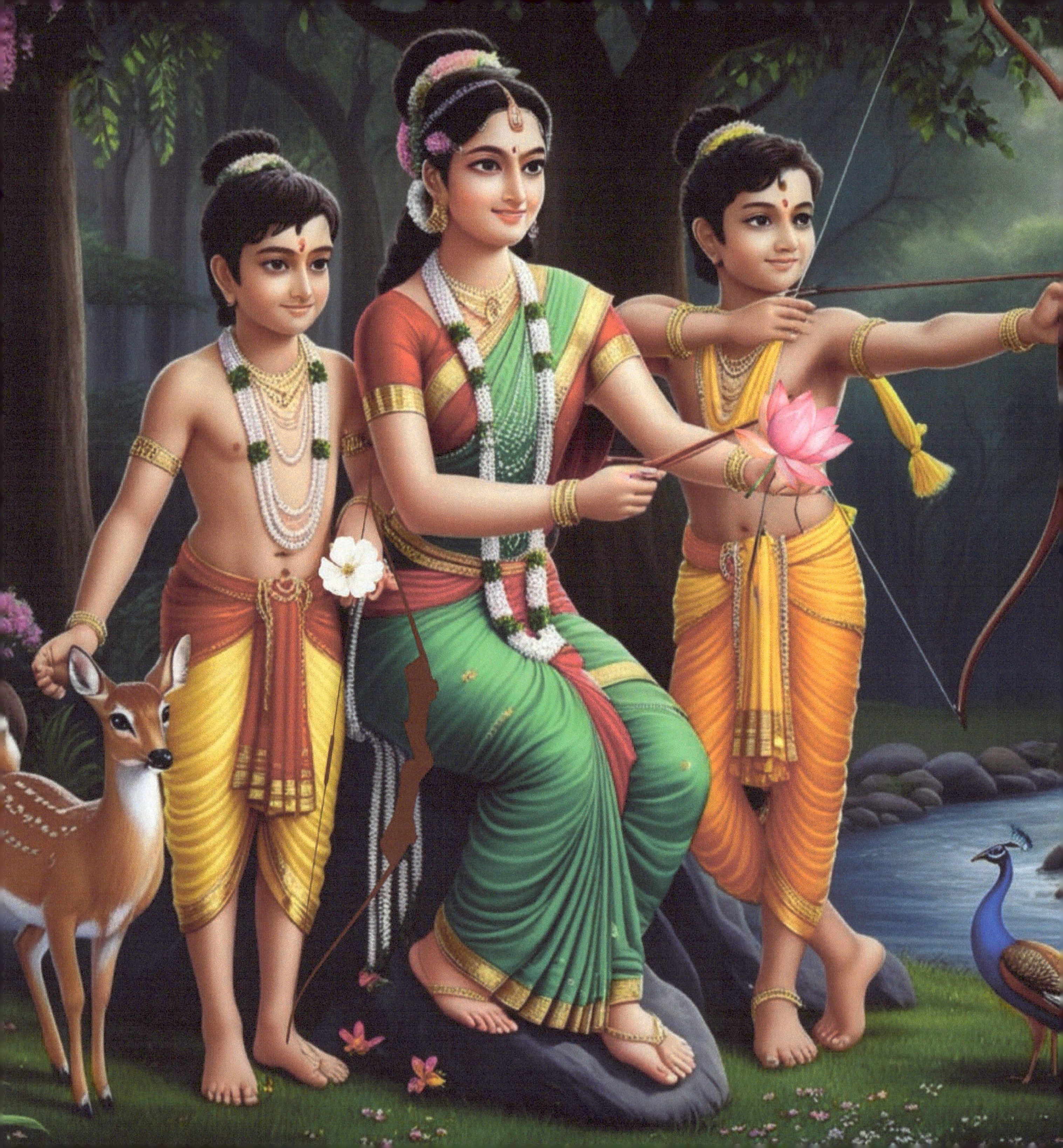

12. Sowing Hope

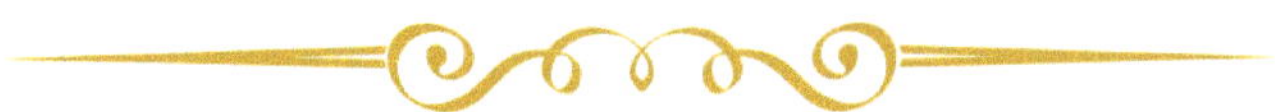

The story of Sita's birth is both miraculous and supernatural. Janaka, king of Mithila, famously known as Rajarshi (Raj=King, Rishi=Sage), was ploughing fields when he discovered a furrow carrying a majestic newborn girl. He adopted her and named her Sita, derived from the Sanskrit word "Seet," meaning furrow. Sita is also affectionately known as Janaki (daughter of Janaka) and Maithili (daughter of the king of Mithila).

As a child, Sita demonstrated extraordinary strength when she effortlessly lifted Lord Shiva's bow, Pinaka, during a playful moment. Janaka was astonished, for it typically took several strong men to move that bow. Realising that Sita was no ordinary child, he cherished her uniqueness.

When Sita reached marriageable age, she married Lord Rama, a union celebrated by all. Their love story took a dramatic turn when Sita renounced the comforts of palace life to join Rama in a fourteen-year exile, showcasing her unwavering devotion as a wife. Tragedy struck when she was abducted by the demon king Ravana. Rama valiantly fought to rescue her, culminating in the fierce battle that restored their love. To prove her purity after her rescue, Sita underwent Agni Pariksha, an ordeal by fire.

Upon returning to Ayodhya, Rama ascended the throne with Sita by his side as queen. However, whispers of doubt began to circulate among the citizens about Sita's chastity. Despite his profound love and trust, Rama made the painful decision to ask Sita to leave the palace for the sake of his kingdom's moral integrity.

A woman needs the most love, care, and attention when she is pregnant, yet Sita was abandoned and left to wander in the jungle while she was pregnant. Rishi Valmiki offered her refuge, and she started living in Rishi's ashrama where Rama's memories continued to haunt and devastate her. The Rishi consoled her, saying, "Sita, if you remain miserable, with a restless mind, then it's going to influence the emotional climate of the unborn children." Taking a deep breath, she gathered her courage, cleared her head, and directed her thoughts to the future of her babies.

In due course, Sita gave birth to twin boys, Luv and Kusha, whom she raised as a devoted single mother. Transforming her grief into a source of strength, Sita nurtured her children with unwavering faith, love, and hope. Luv and Kusha grew into vigilant, valorous, and virtuous young men, reflecting Sita's immense sacrifice and dedication.

When the twins eventually reunited with their father, Lord Rama, Sita chose not to return to Ayodhya. Protecting her self-respect and dignity, she made the ultimate sacrifice by seeking refuge in the embrace of Mother Earth. With a dramatic flourish, the earth split open, and Devi Sita descended, finding peace at last.

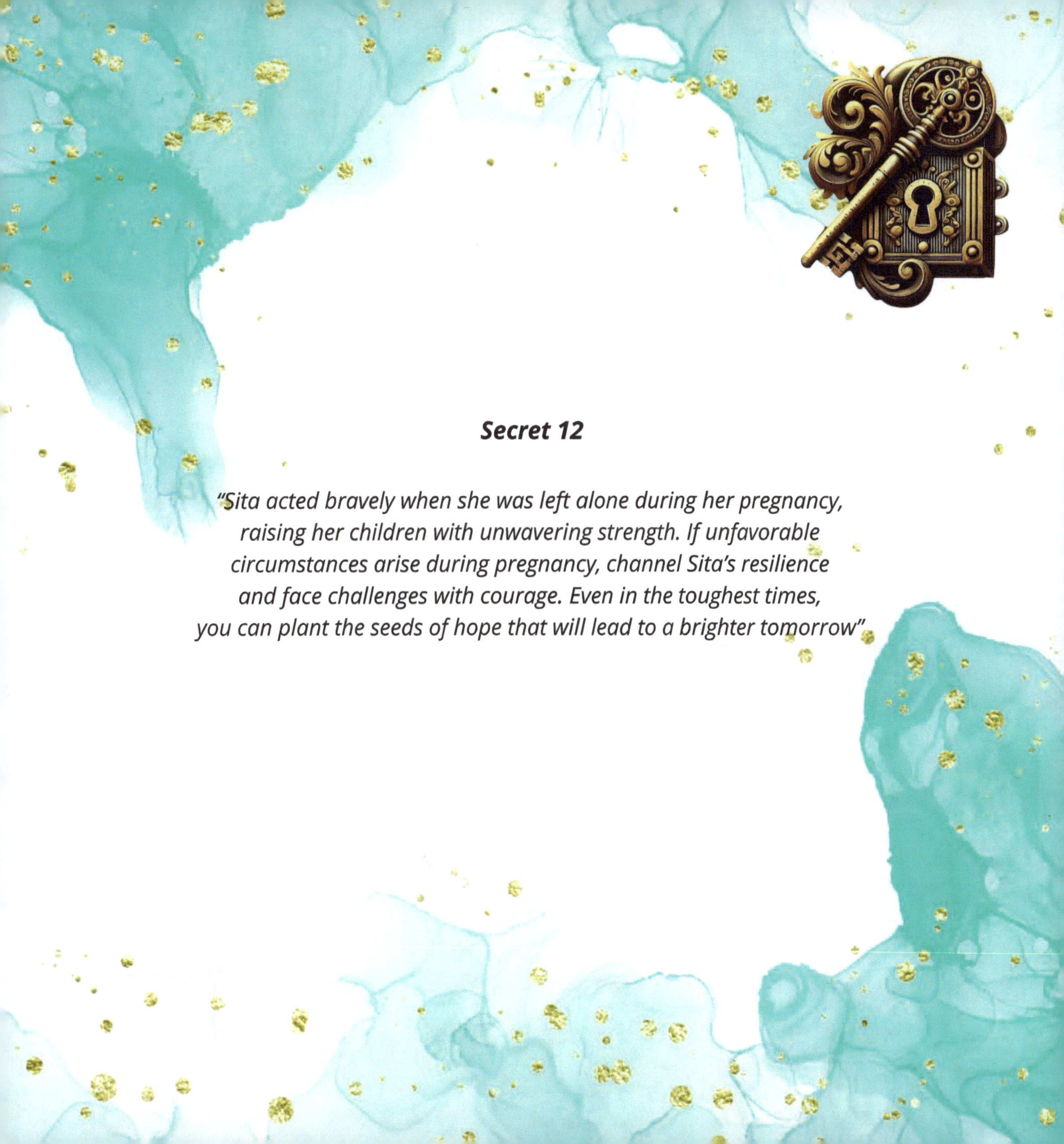

Secret 12

"Sita acted bravely when she was left alone during her pregnancy, raising her children with unwavering strength. If unfavorable circumstances arise during pregnancy, channel Sita's resilience and face challenges with courage. Even in the toughest times, you can plant the seeds of hope that will lead to a brighter tomorrow"

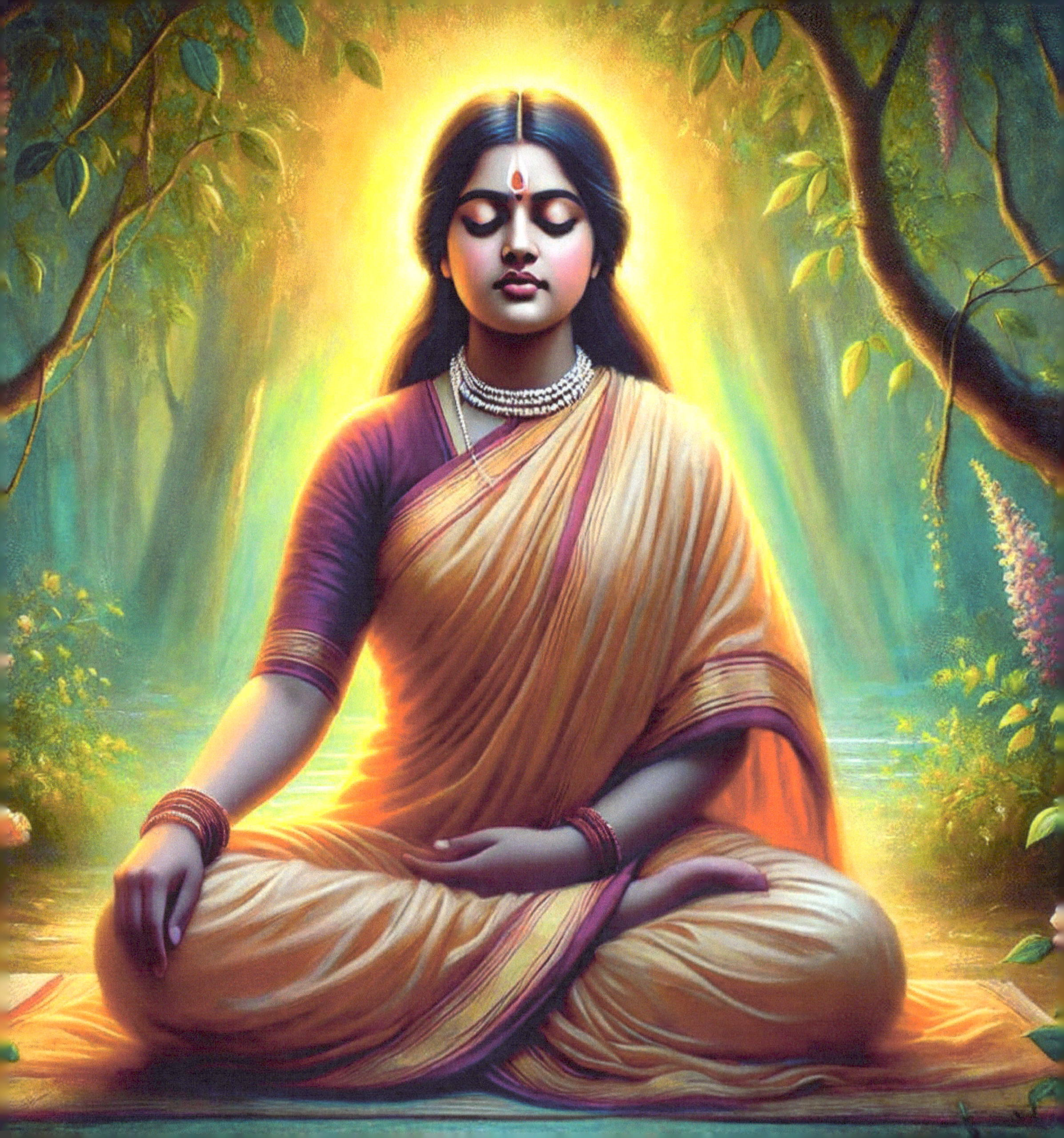

13. Spiritual Preparation

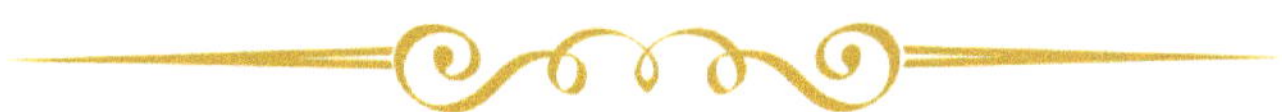

Bhuvaneshwari Devi was the only child of her parents, who were very well-known in northern Calcutta. Bhuvaneshwari Devi was extremely beautiful despite her diminutive stature. At the tender age of 10, she married Shri Vishwanath Datta, who was 16 and already making a mark as a successful attorney with significant societal influence.

Together, Bhuvaneshwari and Vishwanath welcomed 4 sons and 6 daughters into their family. However, tragedy struck when their first son and second daughter passed away in infancy. The following 3 offspring were female. Bhuvaneshwari Devi had a deep desire for a son. Being deeply religious in temperament and a sincere devotee of Lord Shiva, she asked her aunt from Varanasi to make necessary offerings and prayers to Vireshwar Shiva so that a son might be born to her. Meanwhile, she spent her days fasting, meditating, and praying, often practising silence as a form of devotion.

One night, she had a vivid dream in which she felt the divine power of Shiva enter her womb. Awakening with a profound sense of blessing, she knew her prayers had been answered. After some time, on 12 January 1863, she gave birth to a son, whom she named Narendra.

Bhuvaneshwari Devi possessed an exceptional memory and a melodious voice, often reciting entire sections of the Ramayana and Mahabharata from memory. She instilled the moral values of these epics in her children, emphasising the importance of truth, virtue, dignity, and compassion. As a devoted wife, she shared the joys and sorrows of life alongside Vishwanath. She was also a very good wife and companion, sharing joys and sorrows, ups and downs.

Tragedy struck again in February 1884 when her husband passed away unexpectedly. Despite the emotional turmoil, Bhuvaneshwari exhibited remarkable patience, strength, and adaptability in the face of adversity. The relatives who lived on her husband's charity did not help her and deprived her of her possessions. Even then, she performed all her duties with poise and calmness.

Her inclination towards spirituality, serene nature, and sharp intellect is reflected in her son Narendra, who gained fame as Swami Vivekananda. As a young boy, he excelled academically and engaged in various physical pursuits, including sports, gymnastics, wrestling, and bodybuilding. He was a voracious reader, exploring both Hindu scriptures like the Bhagavad Gita and Upanishads, and Western philosophy, history, and spirituality.

He was a major force in the revival of Hinduism in India. He is perhaps best known for his speech which began with the words "Sisters and brothers of America..." in which he introduced Hinduism at the Parliament of the World's Religions in Chicago in 1893. Vivekananda says, "I am indebted to my mother for the efflorescence of my knowledge."

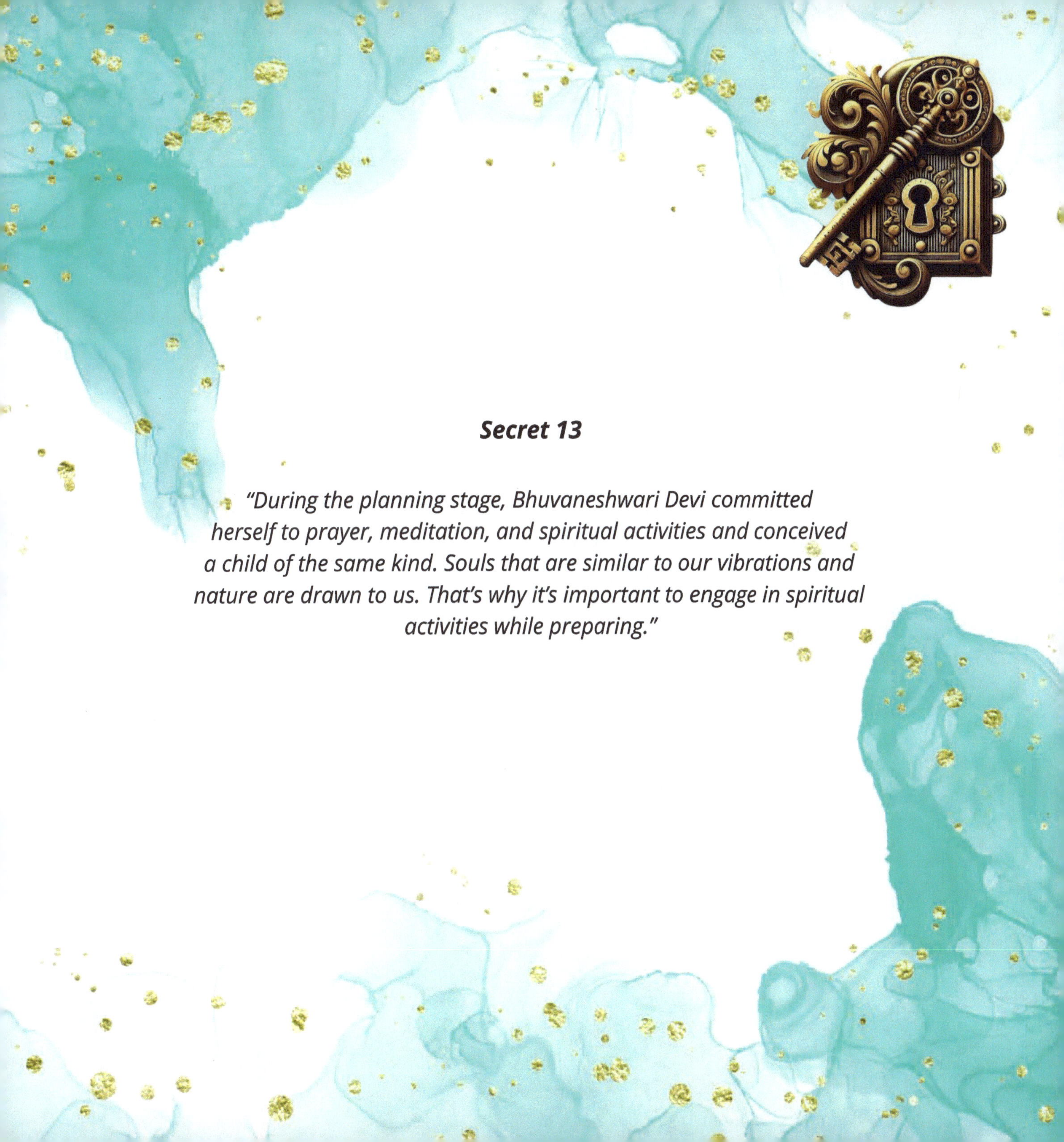

Secret 13

"During the planning stage, Bhuvaneshwari Devi committed herself to prayer, meditation, and spiritual activities and conceived a child of the same kind. Souls that are similar to our vibrations and nature are drawn to us. That's why it's important to engage in spiritual activities while preparing."

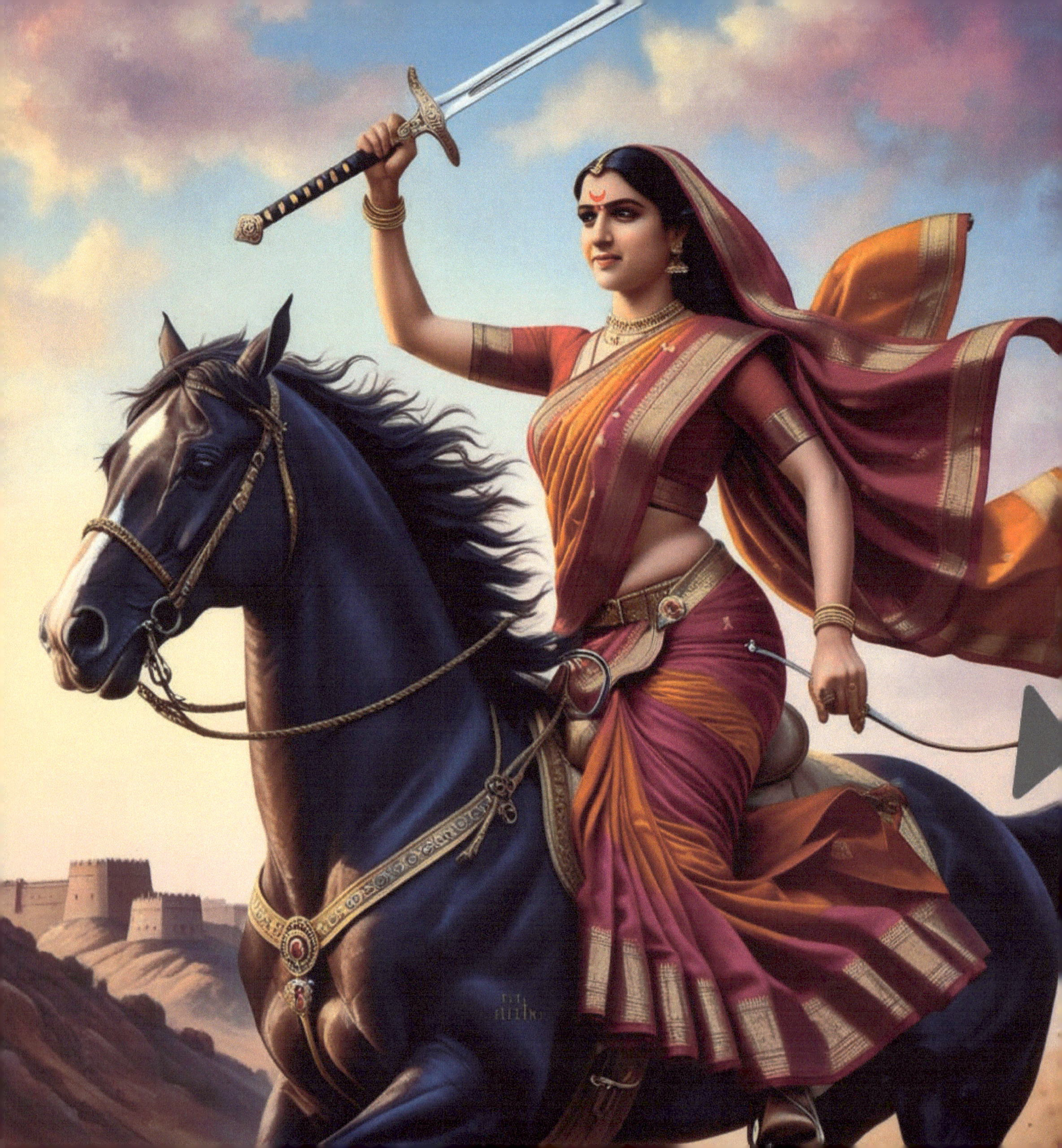

14. Mother's Vision

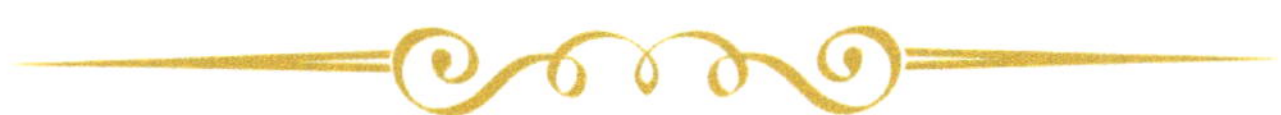

Rajmata Jijabai, affectionately known as Jijau, or JijaMata, is one of India's most inspirational figures. Born on January 12, 1598, in Sindhkhed, Maharashtra, she was the daughter of Mahalasabai and the eminent Sardar Lakhuji Jadhav. From a young age, Jijau witnessed Yavan rulers (Mughals, Nizams, and Adil Shah) abusing people, assaulting women, and demolishing temples. Meanwhile, many Marathas, despite having the strength to challenge the Mughals, chose to serve them in pursuit of wealth and power. Seeing this, Jijau developed a great hatred towards the Yavans.

At the age when other girls were playing with dolls, she preferred to learn sword fighting and horse riding. Her mother nurtured her courage by sharing tales of valour, planting the seeds of strength and resolve in Jijau from an early age.

In 1650, Jijabai was married to Shahaji Bhosle, the son of Maloji Shiledar, at a relatively young age. She quickly realised that though her father and husband were very brave, they were not beneficial to the community as they were serving rulers like the Mughals, Adils, and Nijam. This disheartened Jijau as she was envisioning **Hindavi Swarajya**, the land where people could live with dignity and freedom, a land where women are treated with respect, a land where justice and peace reside.

Jijau strongly desired a son who would rise against the Yavan rulers and fight against injustice. She prayed to Goddess Bhawani for a son who would be wise, brave, fearless, and capable of leading the Marathas in the establishment of Swarajya. Remarkably, Jijau may be the only woman in history who envisioned her child's mission and qualities before his birth. Throughout her pregnancy, she dreamt of wielding a sword, riding a tiger, and slaying enemies—symbols of the Dharmik war.

On 19 February 1630, at Shivneri Fort, Jijau gave birth to Shivaji. Jijau instilled strong values in him from an early age using the wonderful tool of storytelling. She taught him the art of politics and diplomacy through the stories of Krishna. Through Mahabharata tales, little Shivaji learned the importance of fighting against evil to uphold Dharma, while the Ramayana taught him patience, courage, and equality. Chanakya's lessons of strategy and leadership further shaped his understanding of governance and warfare.

Jijau personally supervised Shivaji's training, ensuring he mastered various weapons and military skills. Her unwavering guidance and teachings were instrumental in shaping Shivaji into a valiant and wise leader. Thanks to her influence, Shivaji Raje was able to extricate himself safely from incidents like Afzalkhan's defeat, escape from Agra, etc. Most importantly, under her guidance, Shivaji Raje succeeded in overthrowing centuries of Muslim rule and establishing Hindavi Swarajya, fulfilling the vision Jijau had long dreamt off.

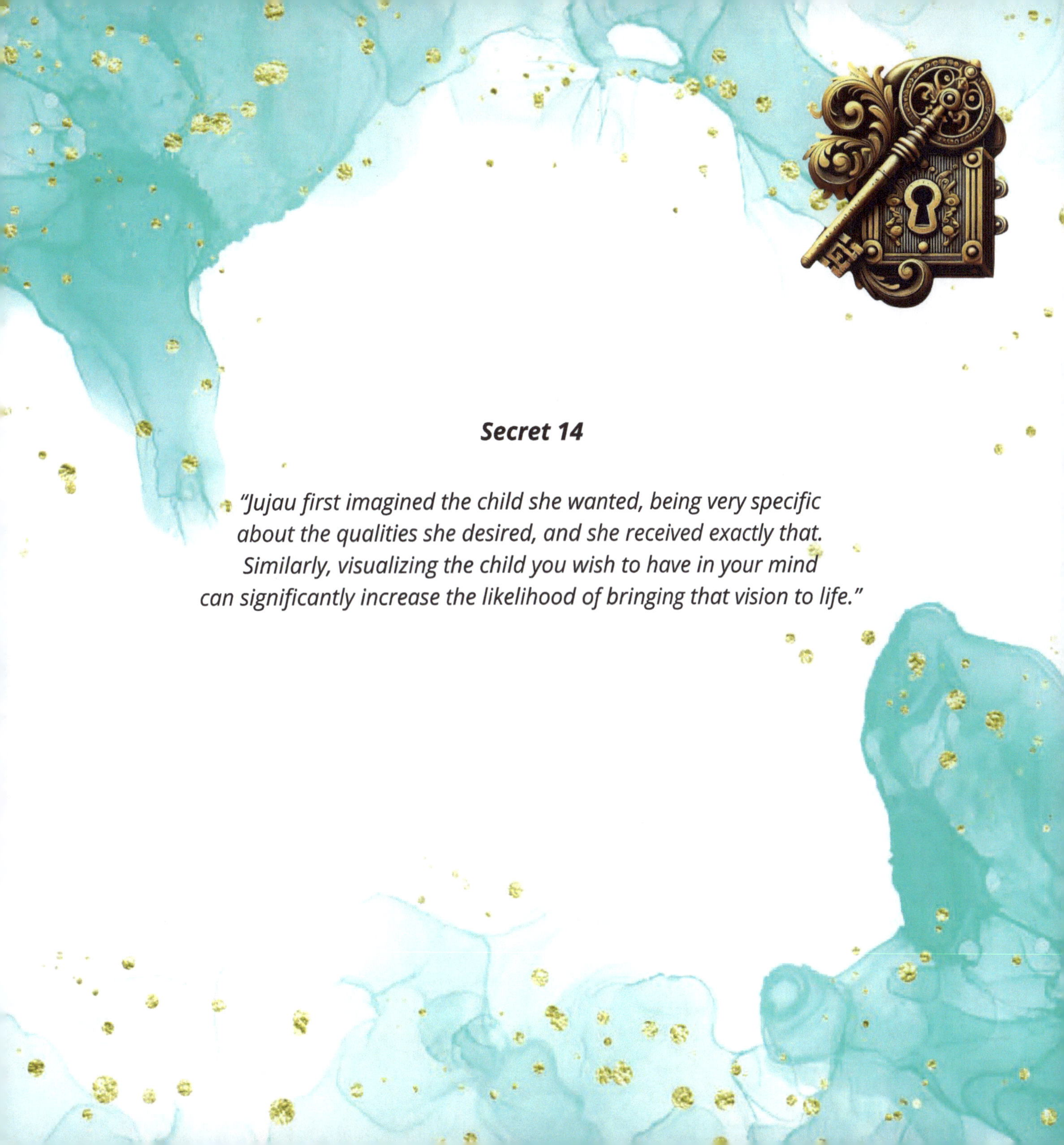

Secret 14

"Jujau first imagined the child she wanted, being very specific about the qualities she desired, and she received exactly that. Similarly, visualizing the child you wish to have in your mind can significantly increase the likelihood of bringing that vision to life."

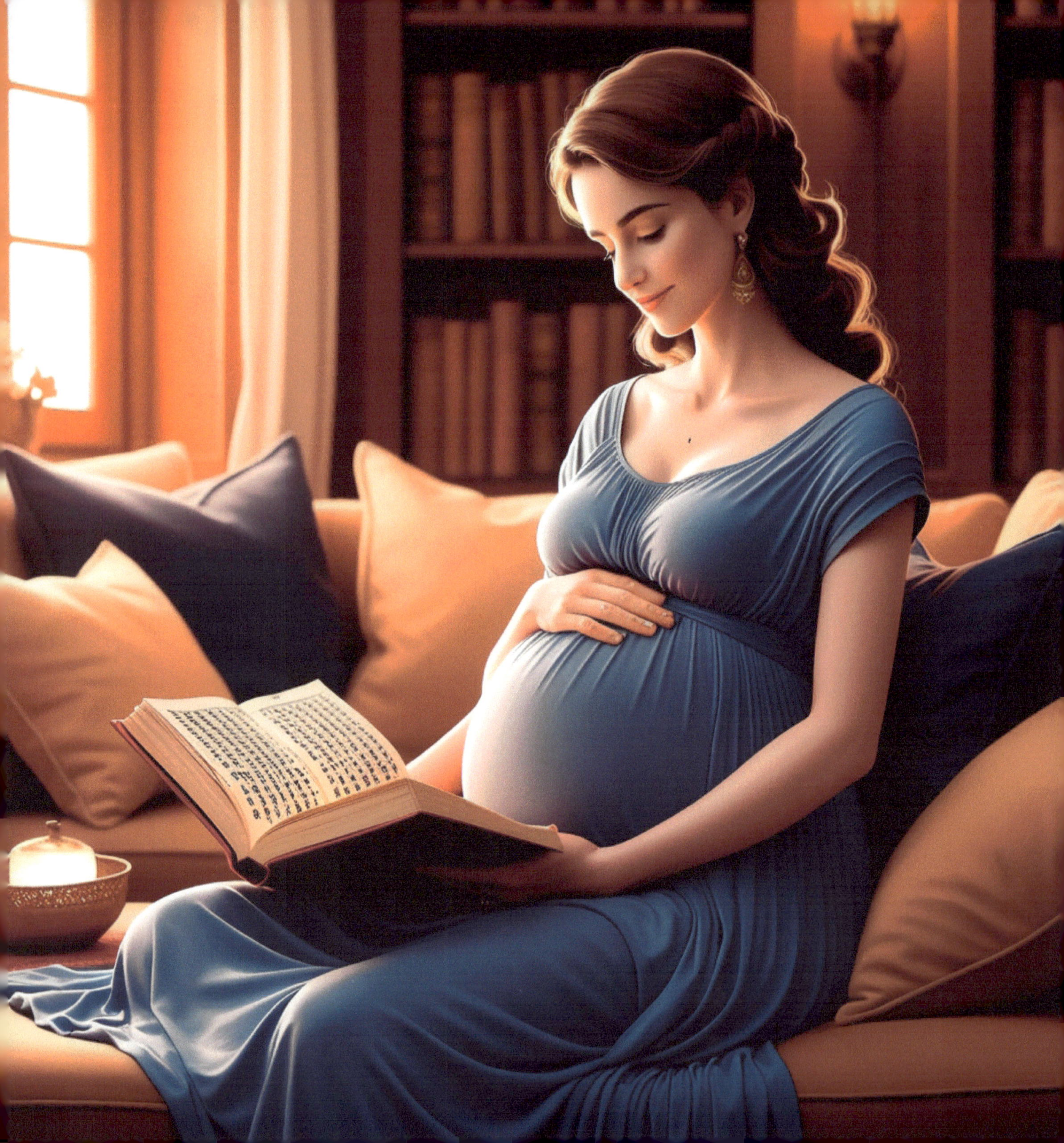

15. Designing Destiny

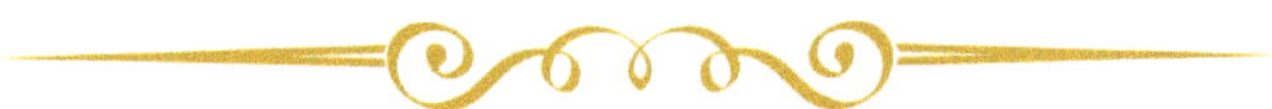

Gabriella's journey into the world of spirituality and Sanskrit language began long before she was born. Her parents, avid travellers with a deep spiritual inclination, were captivated by the diversity and cultural richness of India during one of their visits. They fell in love with India and developed a deep appreciation for the ancient language, Sanskrit.

During her pregnancy, Gabriella's mother decided to delve deeper into this ancient wisdom by enrolling in Sanskrit classes. She would chant and practice writing the Devanagari script, exposing her unborn daughter to the sacred sounds of mantras and prayers. In a way, Gabriella's first introduction to the world was through the vibrations of these ancient Sanskrit chants—her mother's womb became her first classroom.

Growing up, Gabriella was also exposed to the sacred verses of the Bhagavad Gita and the Upanishads. At the tender age of 4, she began formally learning Sanskrit. One of her earliest memories of life is hearing her teacher, Mr. Warwick Jessup, fervently recite the Shiva Sutras in the school assembly every morning. These moments, she says, left an indelible mark on her soul, deepening her connection to the language.

Years later, Gabriella pursued her passion for Sanskrit at the prestigious University of Oxford, where she studied Sanskrit and India's most ancient Hindu philosophical texts, including its great epics, the Ramayana, and the Mahabharata. Though deeply inspired by these epic tales, Gabriella was not sure what direction her life should take after graduation. She explored different paths—composing musicals, performing stand-up comedy, and teaching piano to children. Yet, none of these pursuits felt quite right.

In a twist of fate, she began teaching Sanskrit at a yoga school. It was here that she decided to share her love for Sanskrit online. A simple YouTube video expressing her passion for the language became a turning point. Her focus shifted completely to Sanskrit chanting. One of her videos, on "Madalas Stotram", garnered 2.8 million views, touching the hearts of many with its pure devotion.

So immersed is she in the world of the divine language of India that Gabriella chose to rename herself "Gaiea Sanskrit." 'Gaiea' in Sanskrit means 'to be sung.' For Gaiea Sanskrit itself is music that vibrates with divine sounds. She explains, "The sounds of the Sanskrit language can awaken our souls. It has the capacity to be super comic or super poetic and it is a language that taps into our core."

Gaiea regularly visits India to study music and Sanskrit. Today, she continues to teach Sanskrit, practice the Alexander Technique, and lead Vedic chanting and kirtan sessions. Through her music, she hopes to share the transcendent beauty of Sanskrit with the world.

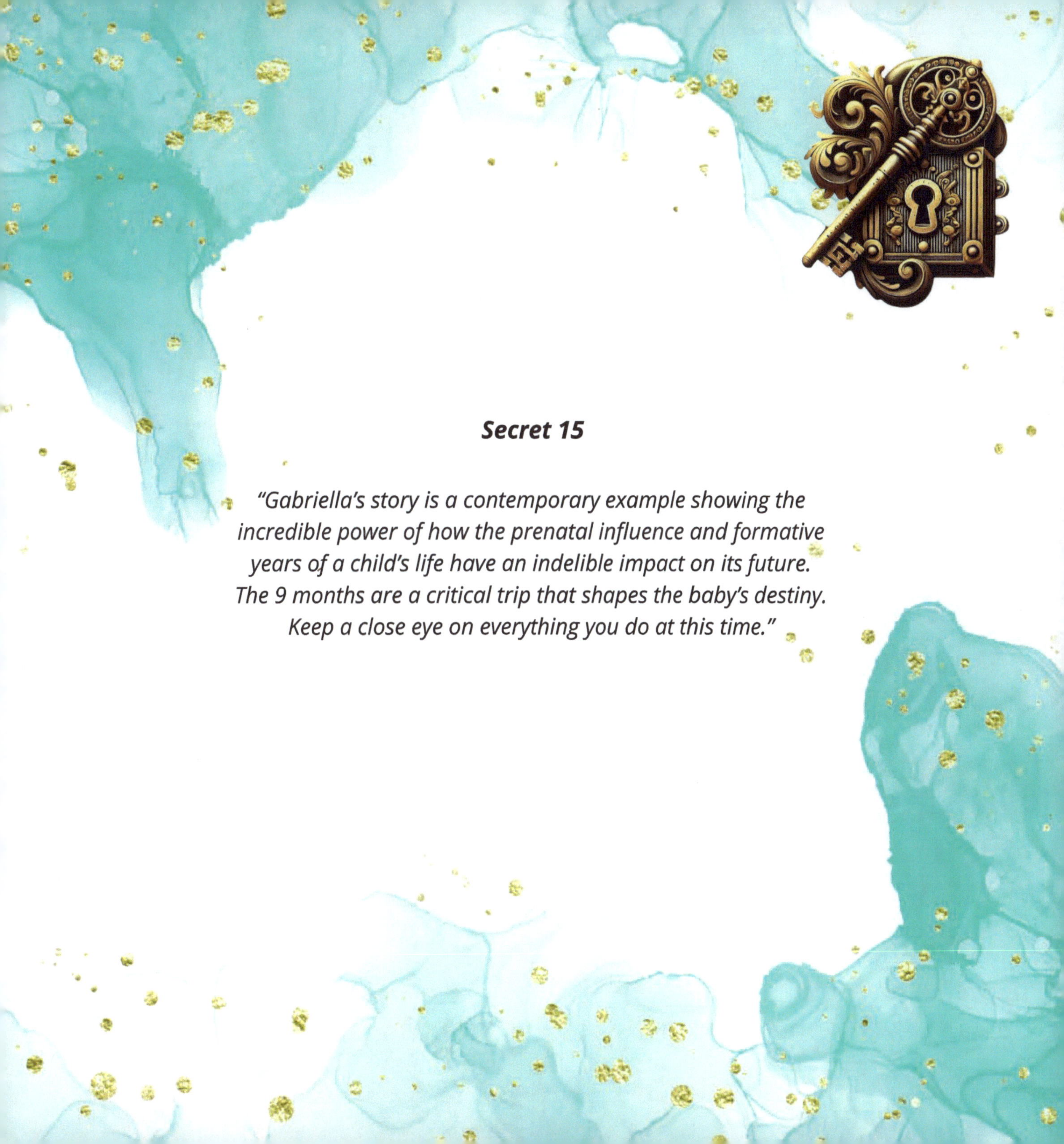

Secret 15

"Gabriella's story is a contemporary example showing the incredible power of how the prenatal influence and formative years of a child's life have an indelible impact on its future. The 9 months are a critical trip that shapes the baby's destiny. Keep a close eye on everything you do at this time."

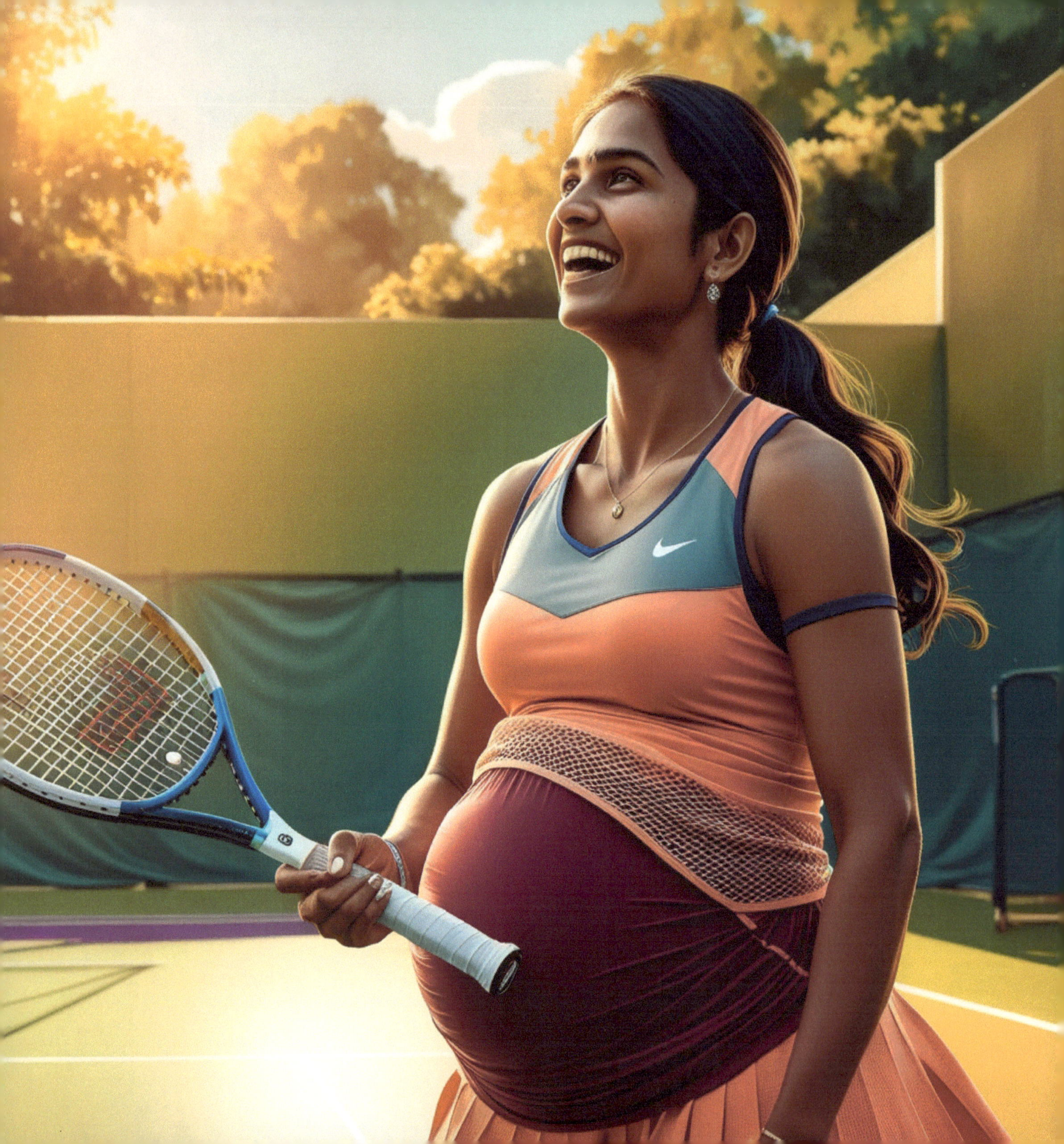

16. Embracing Passion

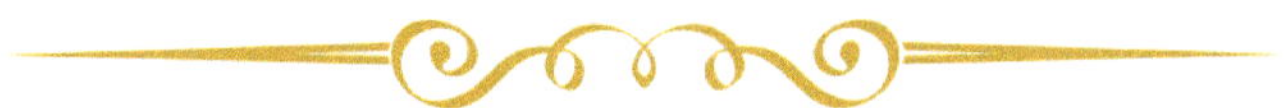

Harvind Singh and Usha Rani, a happily married couple, have one thing in common: a love for sports. Harvind Singh, who holds a PhD in agricultural science, worked at Chaudhary Charan Singh Haryana Agricultural University where his exceptional athletic abilities made him one of the university's standout players. Usha was also a state-level badminton player during her younger days, but as fate would turn out, she could not reach the national level due to unfavourable conditions.

After marriage, the couple welcomed their first daughter, Abu Chandranshu. After her birth, Usha became an active member of the government clubhouse near their home. She was so passionate about the game that when she was expecting their second daughter, Saina, she continued playing. However, when she was in the fifth month, the doctor pleaded with her to stop playing for safety reasons.

Soon after Saina was born on 17 March 1990, she grew up watching her parents play at the Faculty Club of the Haryana Agricultural University and developed a tremendous fascination for the game. Saina's parents successfully cultivated an inherent love for sports in their children as they led by example. When Saina was 8 years old, her father was promoted and transferred to Hyderabad. Confronted with the difficulties of moving to a new city and a language barrier that made it hard for her to connect with other children, Saina decided to focus her energy on badminton by joining a local academy.

Her parents went above and beyond to support her ambitions. Despite the academy being 25 kilometres from their home, they ensured that Saina's training began at 4 a.m. every day. Their unwavering dedication and determination played a crucial role in helping their daughter pursue her dreams.

After Saina's remarkable talent caught the attention of Mr S.M. Arif, an award-winning badminton coach, her journey took off. At just 14 years old, she won a silver medal at the Commonwealth Youth Games, marking the beginning of her ascent in the sport. By the age of 18, Saina became an integral part of the Indian Badminton squad and a teenage sensation throughout India.

Reflecting on this, Saina's father remarked in an interview with the Hindustan Times, "I believe little Saina absorbed the lessons of badminton in the womb, much like Abhimanyu learned about the Chakravyuh."

Her cap is decorated with feathers from being the first Indian woman to win a Super Series tournament to the first Indian to win the World Junior Badminton Championships and then a medal in Badminton at the Olympics. Saina's remarkable journey, rooted in her family's love for sports, has inspired countless individuals and demonstrated the power of perseverance.

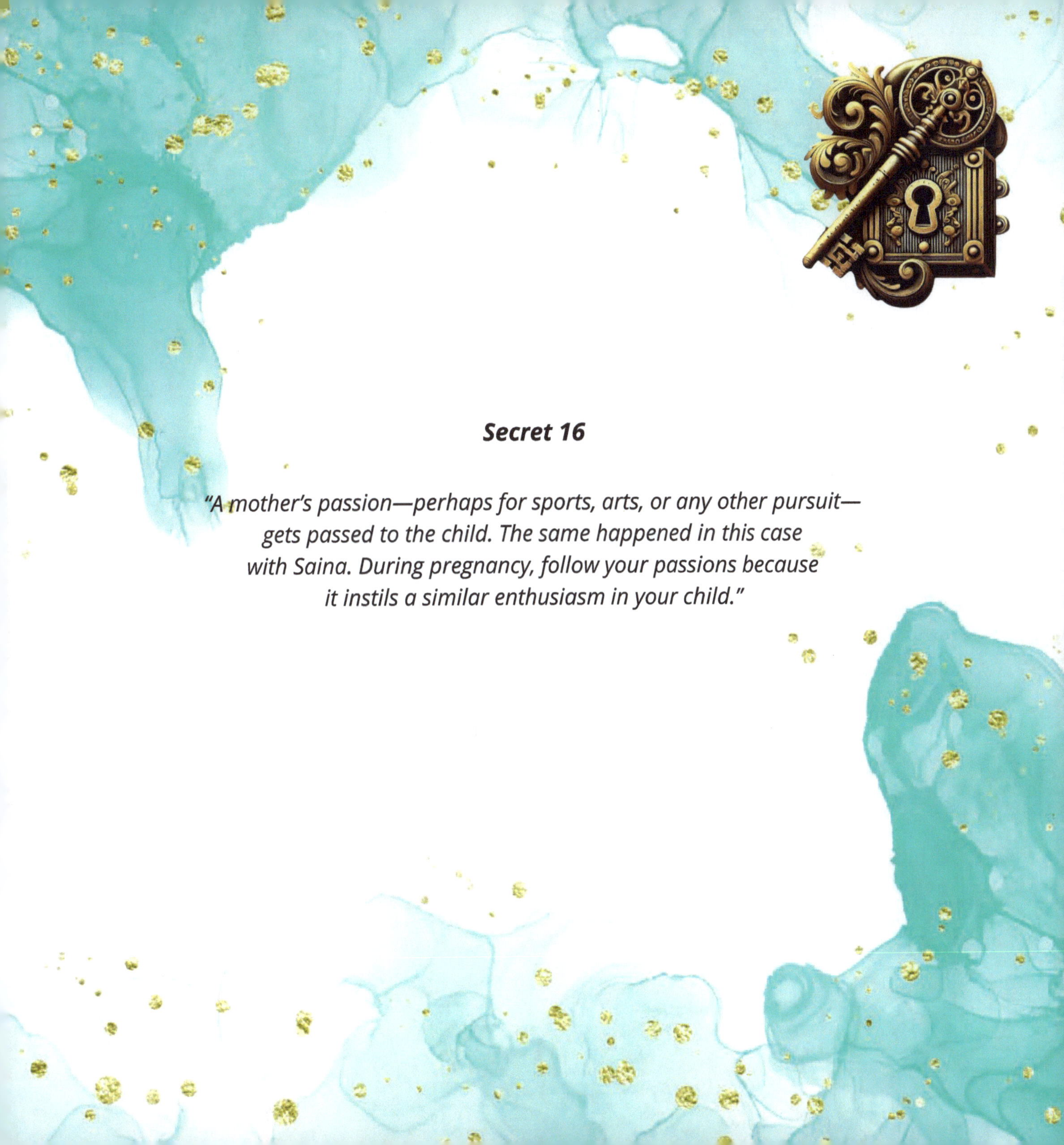

Secret 16

*"A mother's passion—perhaps for sports, arts, or any other pursuit—
gets passed to the child. The same happened in this case
with Saina. During pregnancy, follow your passions because
it instils a similar enthusiasm in your child."*

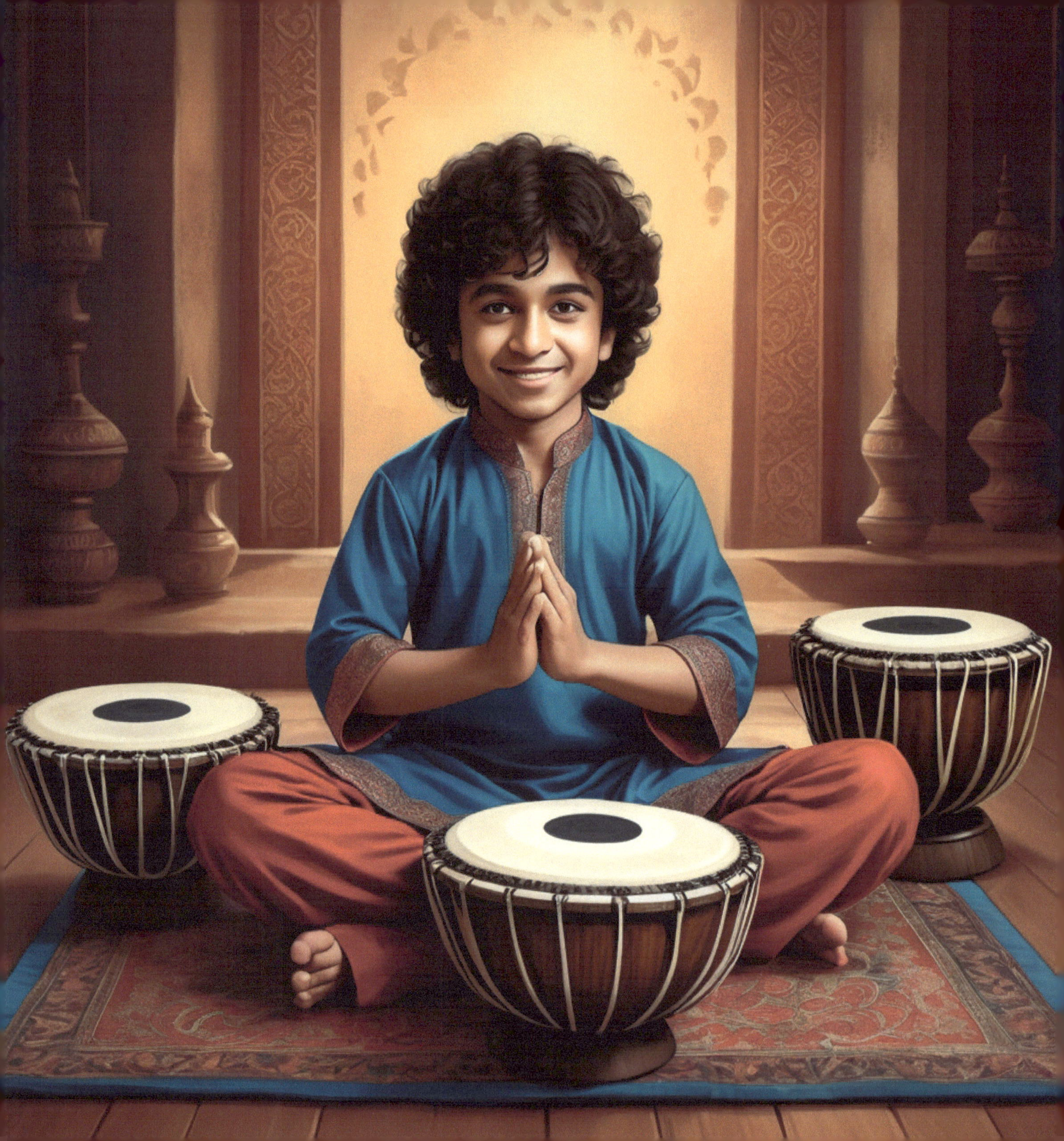

17. Unbreakable Bond

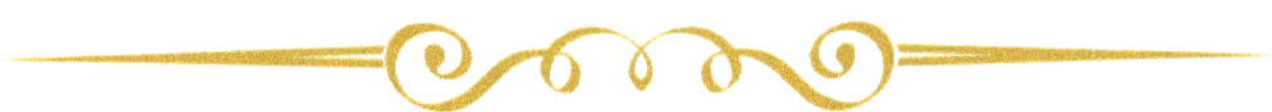

Ustad Alla Rakha was born on April 29, 1919, in the small village of Phagwal, Jammu, as one of 7 children in a humble, poor family. At the age of 8, he heard the Tabla for the first time and became deeply fascinated by the instrument. However, in his family, singing and learning instruments were not encouraged. Driven by his love for music, Alla Rakha made the bold decision to run away from home at the age of 12 to pursue his dreams.

He began his formal training in Tabla under Mian Kader Baksh of the Punjab Gharana and additionally studied classical music and Raag Vidya under Ustad Ashiq Ali Khan of the Patiala Gharana. Through years of patience, dedication, and disciplined practice, Alla Rakha honed his craft. He eventually became a staff artist at All India Radio and even composed music for Bollywood films. However, his most significant contribution was in raising global awareness of Indian classical music and the Tabla, making the instrument known and respected worldwide. He was married to his cousin Bavi Begum, and the couple had 3 sons, Zakir Hussain, Fazal Qureshi, and Taufiq Qureshi; two daughters, Khurshid Aulia and Razia.

Zakir was introduced to Tabla before even he was born. Ustad Alla Rakha used to gently tap Bavi Begam's belly with his fingers while she was expecting Zakir. And those were his first lessons. He heard the Tabla regularly as an unborn child when Alla Rakha used to play it. When Zakir was born, Alla Rakha was critically ill. He was sick with some unknown ailment. After birth, when barely a few minutes old, Zakir was taken to Alla Rakha, his father. He whispered Tabla syllables, "ta tin tin ta," into the baby's ears. He even tied a little Tabla to the baby's crib. Little Zakir used to reach out to the Tabla very eagerly. Alla Rakha also used to put little Zakir on his chest and would play a rhythm gently on his back. As a toddler, Zakir used to attend his father's concert. He grew up in the atmosphere of music 24 hours a day. The Tabla got so ingrained in Zakir's system that before he even learned the Tabla, he knew its language, and he never consciously learned it.

At the age of 7, Zakir gave his first public performance. By 12, he started touring and attained great success at the age of 18. By collaborating with international artists, he has elevated the status of his instrument both in India and globally, bringing the tabla into a new dimension of renown and appreciation. He is the recipient of countless awards and honours including Padma Vibhushan, the Sangeet Natak Akademi Award, the Grammy Award, etc.

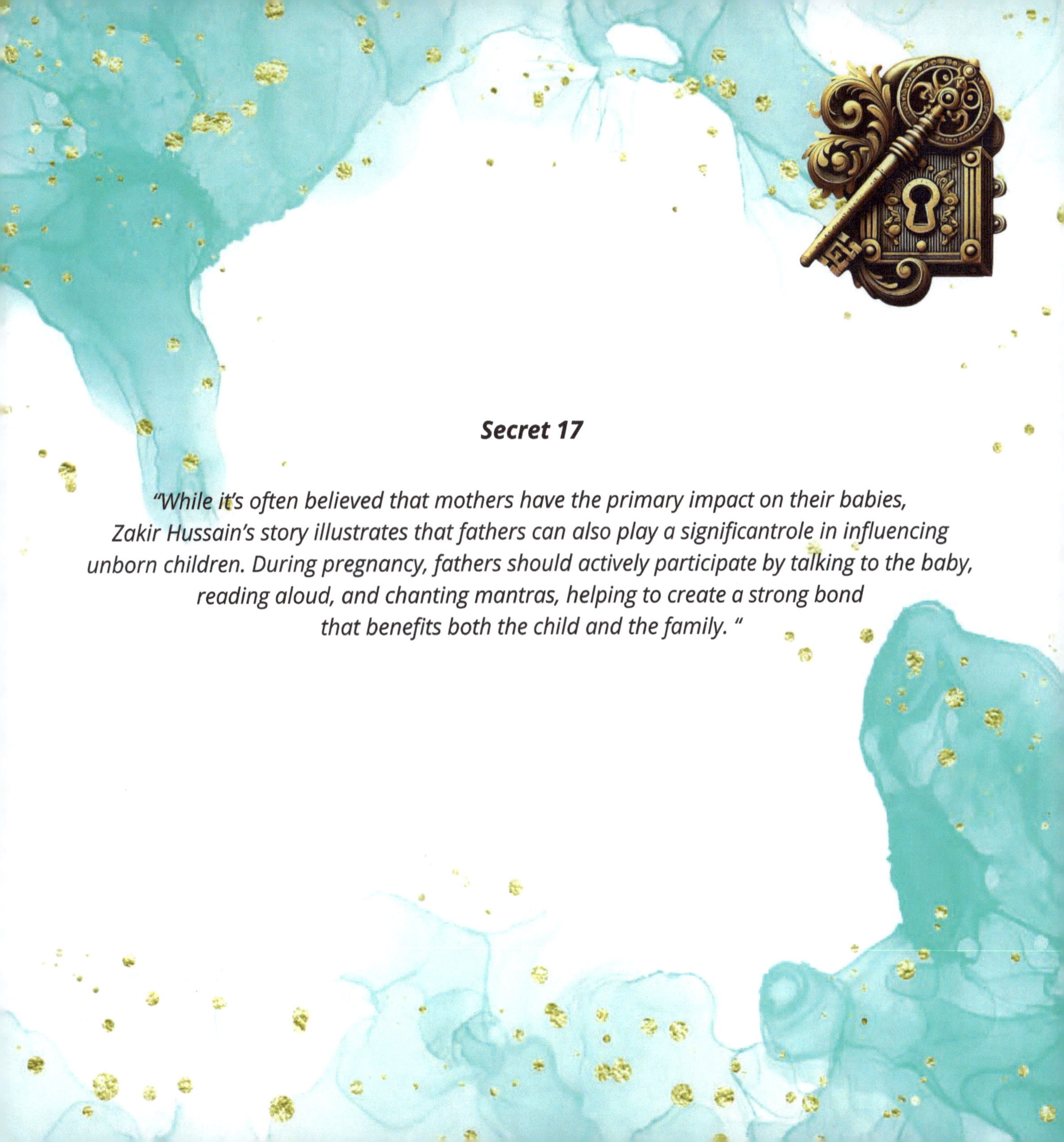

Secret 17

"While it's often believed that mothers have the primary impact on their babies, Zakir Hussain's story illustrates that fathers can also play a significantrole in influencing unborn children. During pregnancy, fathers should actively participate by talking to the baby, reading aloud, and chanting mantras, helping to create a strong bond that benefits both the child and the family. "

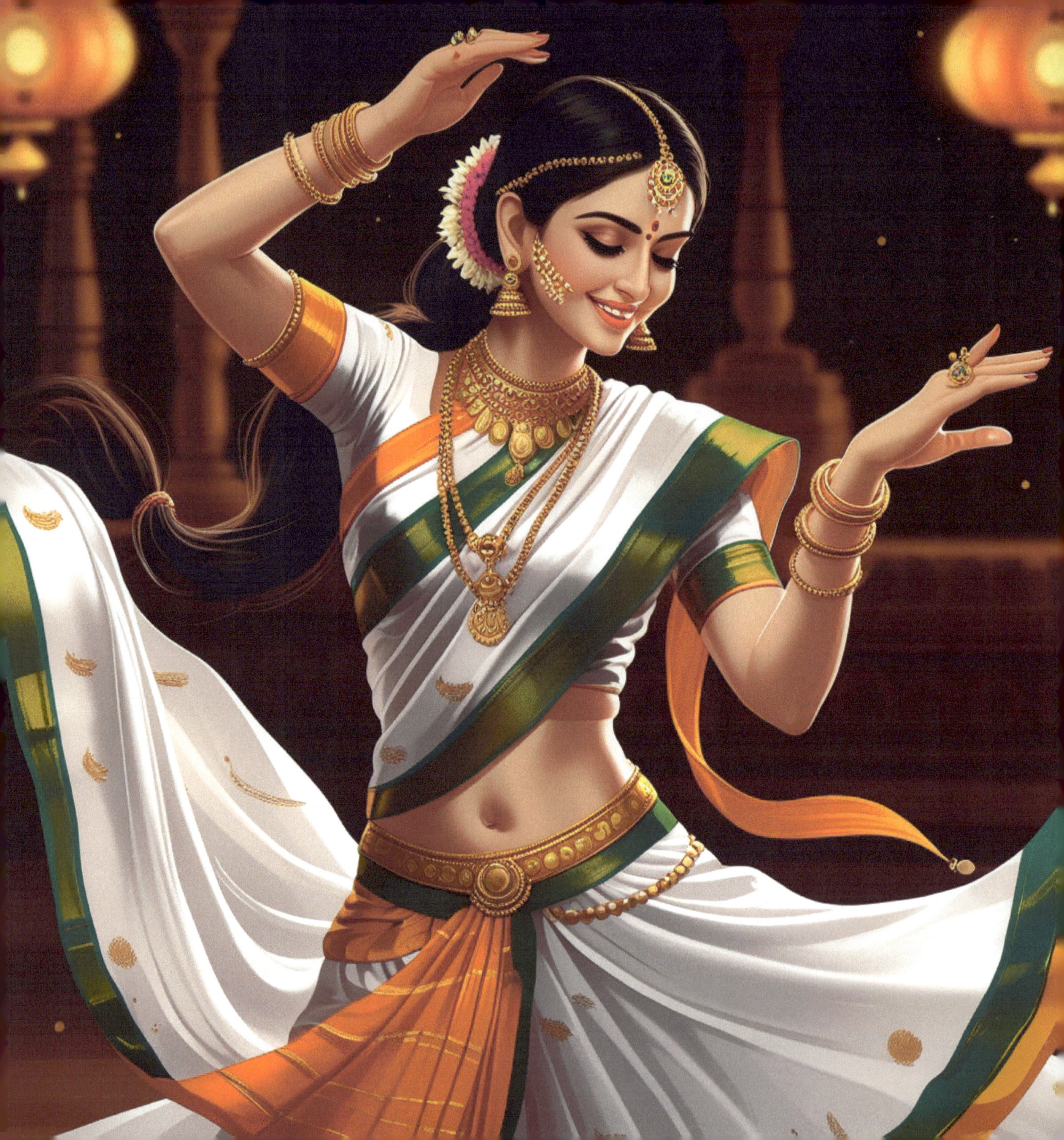

18. Deep Desires

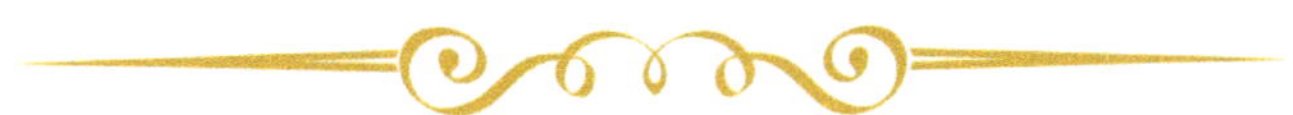

Sonalika Padhi, a renowned Odissi dancer, hails from humble beginnings. From a young age, she exhibited a hardworking, bright, and energetic spirit. With her mother and aunt as classical dancers, Sonalika naturally developed a deep passion for dance. She aspired to pursue a career in Odissi while balancing her academics. However, frequent relocations due to her father's job and the demands of higher studies hindered her from fully committing to dance. Ultimately, she became a scientist and began her career as a Junior Scientist in Lucknow. After 2 years, she married Srimanta Purohit, a supportive software engineer, and settled in Bangalore.

Srimanta being a very supportive husband encouraged her to go back to dancing. Due to his encouragement, Sonalika enrolled in the newly opened Nrityantar Academy of Performing Arts where she met her Guru Madhulita Mohapatra. Even during her pregnancy, she practised diligently. In this way, Shrinika got exposed to the rhythms of music and dance in the womb itself.

Just 2 months after Shrinika's birth, Sonalika resumed her Odissi rehearsals. As a baby, Shrinika delighted in playing with her mother's dance costumes and ghungaroos, often mimicking dance postures and movements as soon as she could stand. Sonalika never wanted her daughter to become an Odissi dancer just because she is one, but observing Shrinika's enthusiasm, she decided to nurture it further. Sonalika began taking Shrinika to the dance studio, where little Shrinika picked up dance poses just by observing and stunned everyone.

At the age of 3 when children do not think of anything beyond toys, Shrinika gave her first performance at our annual Naman Odissi festival in 2013. The audience was captivated by the sight of this doll-like girl on stage. As she danced, her innocence, expressive gestures, and graceful movements enchanted everyone, earning her a standing ovation. Since then, her dance has become everyone's delight and demand. Being a crowd-puller, she has been a regular feature in several major dance events and festivals both at national and international levels. Shrinika is recognised as one of India's 21 young prodigies by esteemed channels like News 18 and CNN and has received numerous accolades, including the Aekalavya Award and Odissi Pratibha. Today, she is affectionately known as the "Wonder Kid of Odissi".

Now 14 years old, Shrinika strikes a remarkable balance between her dance and studies. She assists her mother with household chores and excels in drawing, proving she is poised for a bright future.

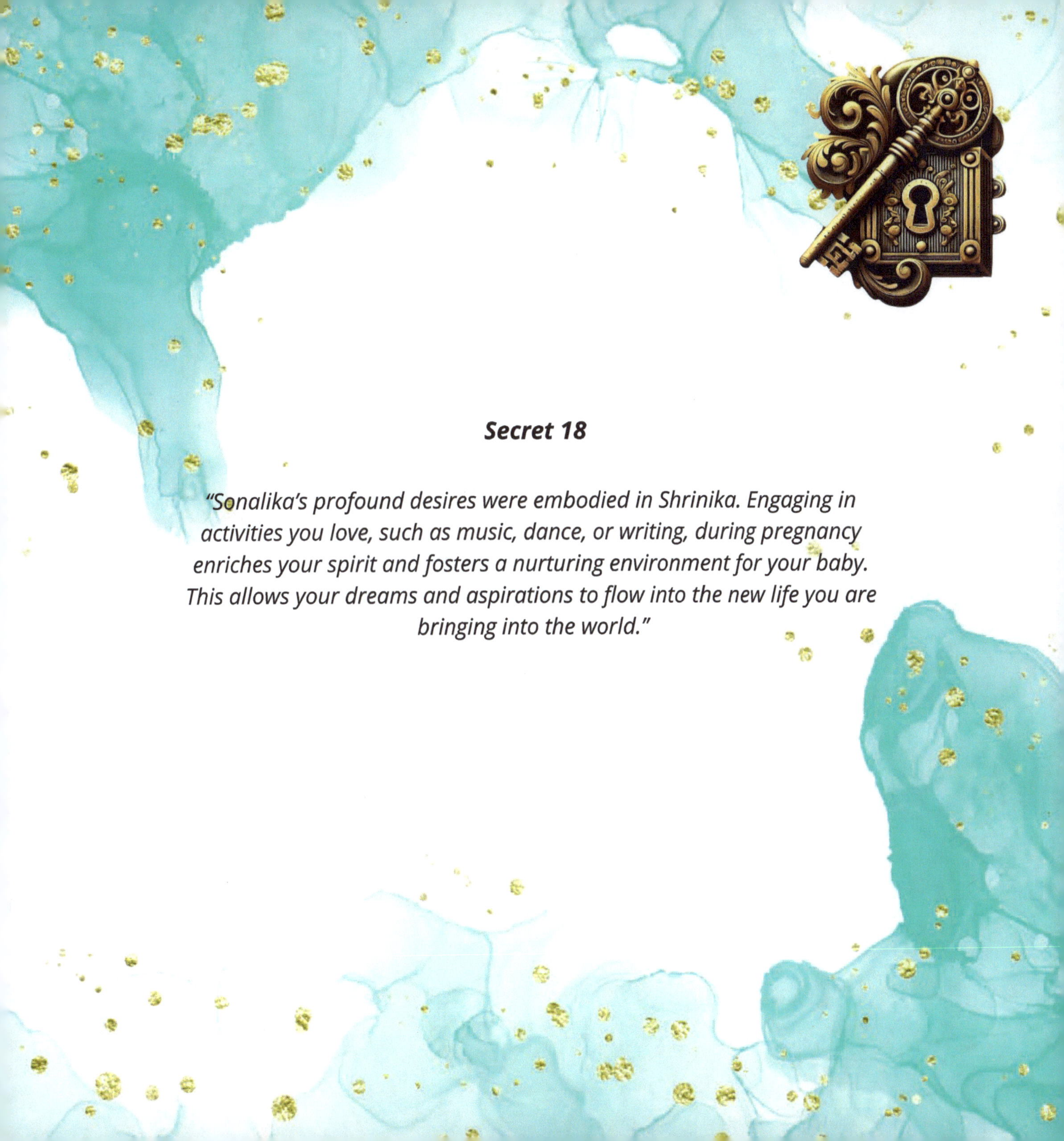

Secret 18

"Sonalika's profound desires were embodied in Shrinika. Engaging in activities you love, such as music, dance, or writing, during pregnancy enriches your spirit and fosters a nurturing environment for your baby. This allows your dreams and aspirations to flow into the new life you are bringing into the world."

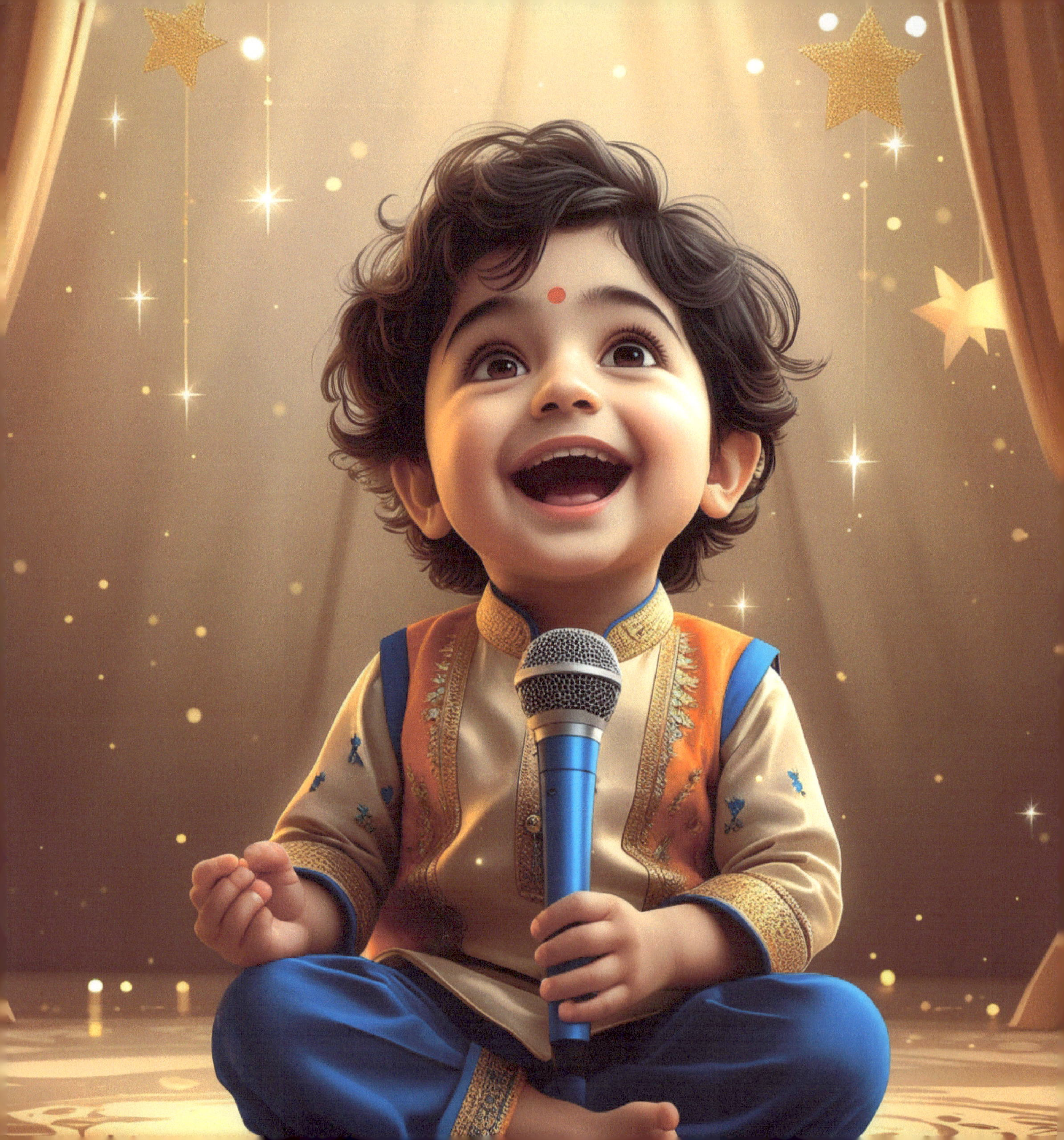

19. The Prenatal Melody

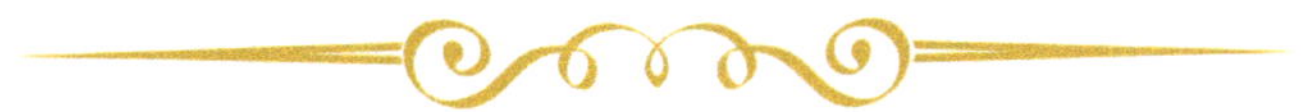

Dinanath Mangeshkar was a renowned Marathi theatre actor, a prominent Natya Sangeet musician, and an exceptional Hindustani classical vocalist. Born on December 29, 1900, in the lush village of Mangeshi, Goa, he was the son of Ganesh Bhat Navathe Hardikar and Yesubai Rane. Blessed with a high, melodious voice, Dinanath began taking music lessons at the tender age of 5. His striking looks and talent quickly gained him popularity in Marathi theatre.

At 21, Dinanath married 19-year-old Shevanti, the daughter of a wealthy Gujarati businessman, Seth Haridas Ramdas Lad, in Thalnar, Maharashtra. Music and theatre rehearsals were a regular part of their household, as Dinanath ran a theatre company that produced musical plays. This environment provided invaluable exposure to music and acting for his wife during pregnancy as they welcomed 5 children Lata, Meena, Asha, Usha, and Hridaynath.

Lata began acting in plays at just 5 years old. One day, Dinanath's disciples Chandrakant and Suryakant were practising raag (a collection of musical notes) while 4–5-year-old Lata was playing nearby. Suddenly, a note of the Raag that they were rendering jarred. This did not go unnoticed by little Lata, and she started correcting them. Observing this, Dinanath recognised his daughter's innate talent, exclaiming to her mother, "We have a singer at home. We never knew it."

Tragically, Dinanath passed away when Lata was only 13, thrusting the financial responsibilities of the family onto her shoulders. Lata started her career in 1942, shortly after her father's death. A family friend, Vinayak Damodar Karnataki, helped her secure acting roles in Marathi and Hindi films. However, her initial years were challenging; she faced numerous rejections from contemporary music composers, who criticised her voice as too thin and sharp for the prevailing musical style. To appease the music directors, she would often imitate famous singers like Noor Jahan.

Lata's breakthrough came with the song "Dil Mera Toda, Mujhe Kahin Ka Na Chhoda" from the 1948 film *Majboor*. Her first major hit was "Ayega Anewala," featured in the 1949 film *Mahal*. From that point on, Lata's music career took off as she started working with all major music directors and playback singers of the time. Her voice became synonymous with the era's most glamorous heroines, from Madhubala to Meena Kumari.

Lata's illustrious career, which began in 1942, spanned over 7 decades. She recorded songs for over a thousand Hindi films and lent her voice to songs in more than 36 regional Indian languages and foreign languages, solidifying her legacy as one of India's greatest musical icons.

Not only did Lata Mangeshkar achieve legendary status, but her siblings—Meena, Asha, Usha, and Hridaynath—also made significant contributions and established their names in the music industry.

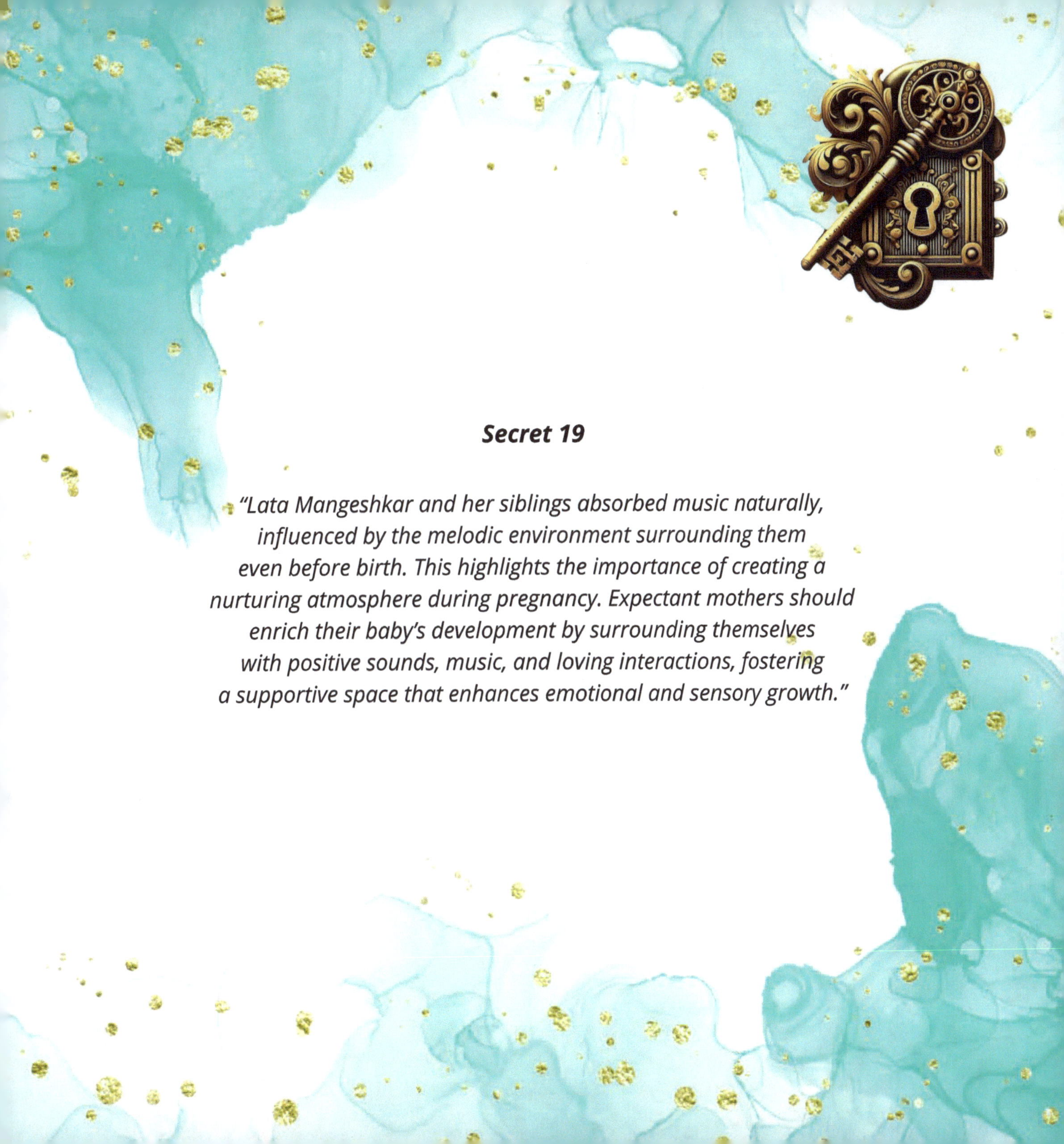

Secret 19

*"Lata Mangeshkar and her siblings absorbed music naturally,
influenced by the melodic environment surrounding them
even before birth. This highlights the importance of creating a
nurturing atmosphere during pregnancy. Expectant mothers should
enrich their baby's development by surrounding themselves
with positive sounds, music, and loving interactions, fostering
a supportive space that enhances emotional and sensory growth."*

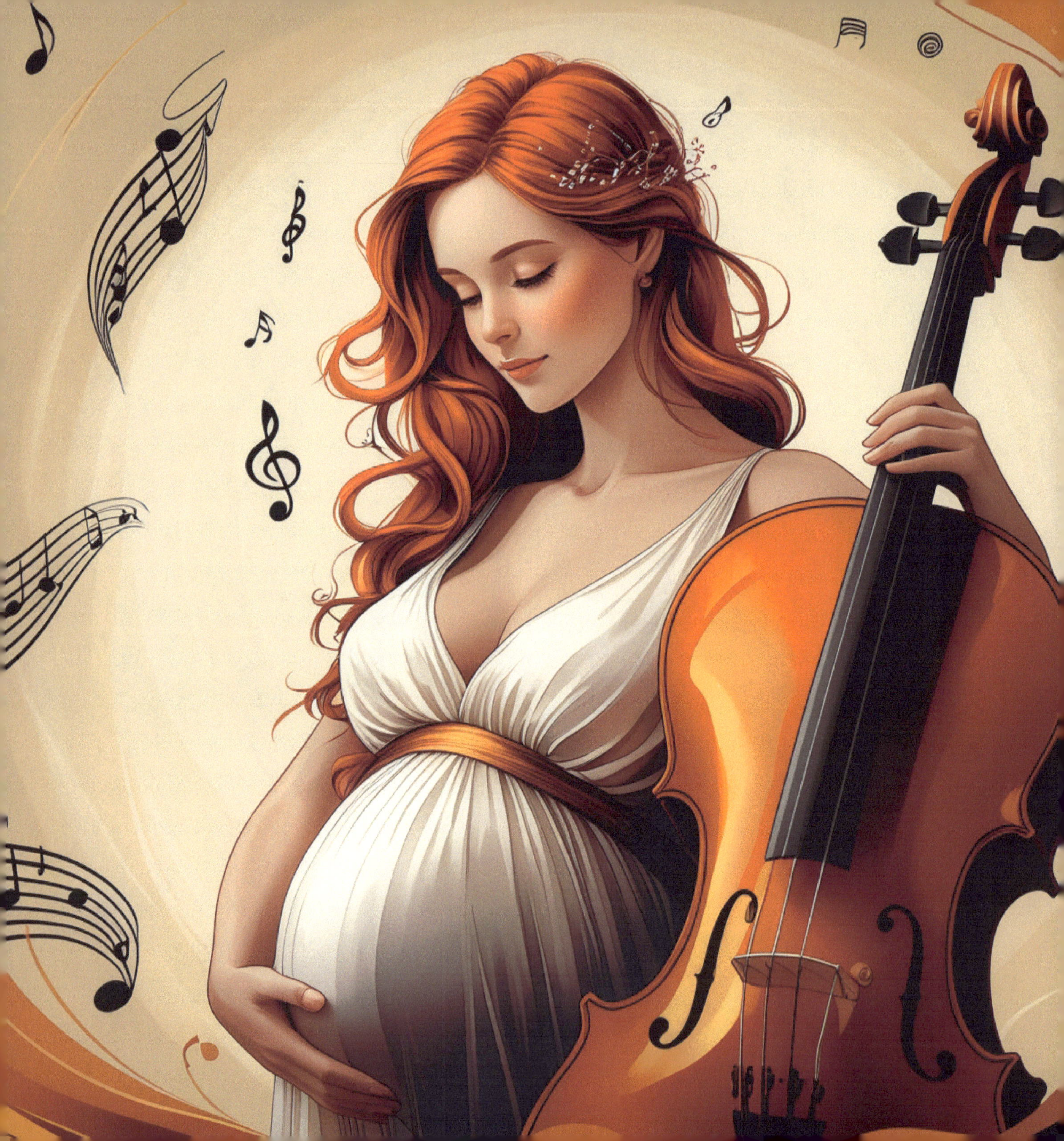

20. The Gift of Sound

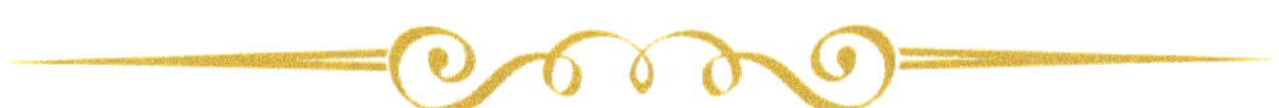

Boris Brott was born on March 14, 1944, to Alexander and Lotte/Charlotte Brott in Montreal, QC. His father, Alexander Brott, was a renowned violinist and composer, while his mother, Charlotte, was a professional cellist. During her pregnancy, Charlotte immersed herself in music, creating several scores for a program, but unfortunately, she never got the chance to perform after that.

From a young age, Boris exhibited a natural curiosity and passion for music. He learned to play the violin under his father's guidance and, at just 5 years old, made his debut performance with the Montreal Symphony Orchestra. His commitment to music led him to enrol in courses at the Conservatoire de musique du Québec and McGill University. Additionally, he further refined his skills in conducting at the Pierre Monteux summer school.

As he practised conducting in his youth, Boris experienced a remarkable phenomenon: he recognised certain music scores related to the cello section without having learned them. He intuitively knew the flow of the pieces before even turning the pages. When he shared these strange mysterious experiences with his mother, she felt intrigued and asked Boris to play them. When he played the scores, it was revealed that they were the same ones Charlotte had composed during her pregnancy. In an extraordinary twist of fate, Boris Brott could recognise and perform the music his mother had practised while carrying him—an incredible testament to the power of prenatal musical exposure.

When Boris was just 14 years old, he won the first prize at the Pan-American conducting competition, and he was unstoppable after that. He earned victories in many competitions like the Liverpool Conductors' Competition in Great Britain and the Dimitri Mitropoulos International Conductors' Competition in New York. His contributions to music education earned him Canada's highest civic honour, the Officer of the Order of Canada.

He authored hundreds of scripts that introduced around 2 million kids to the great composers and instruments of the orchestra and received the National Child Day Award. He also pursued a parallel career as a motivational speaker, delivering 35 presentations annually to Fortune 500 companies around the world, linking music and business. His speeches often emphasised the themes of teamwork and creativity, illustrating the parallels between music and business. Despite his musical success and acclaim, he remained humble and never lost his passion for the art.

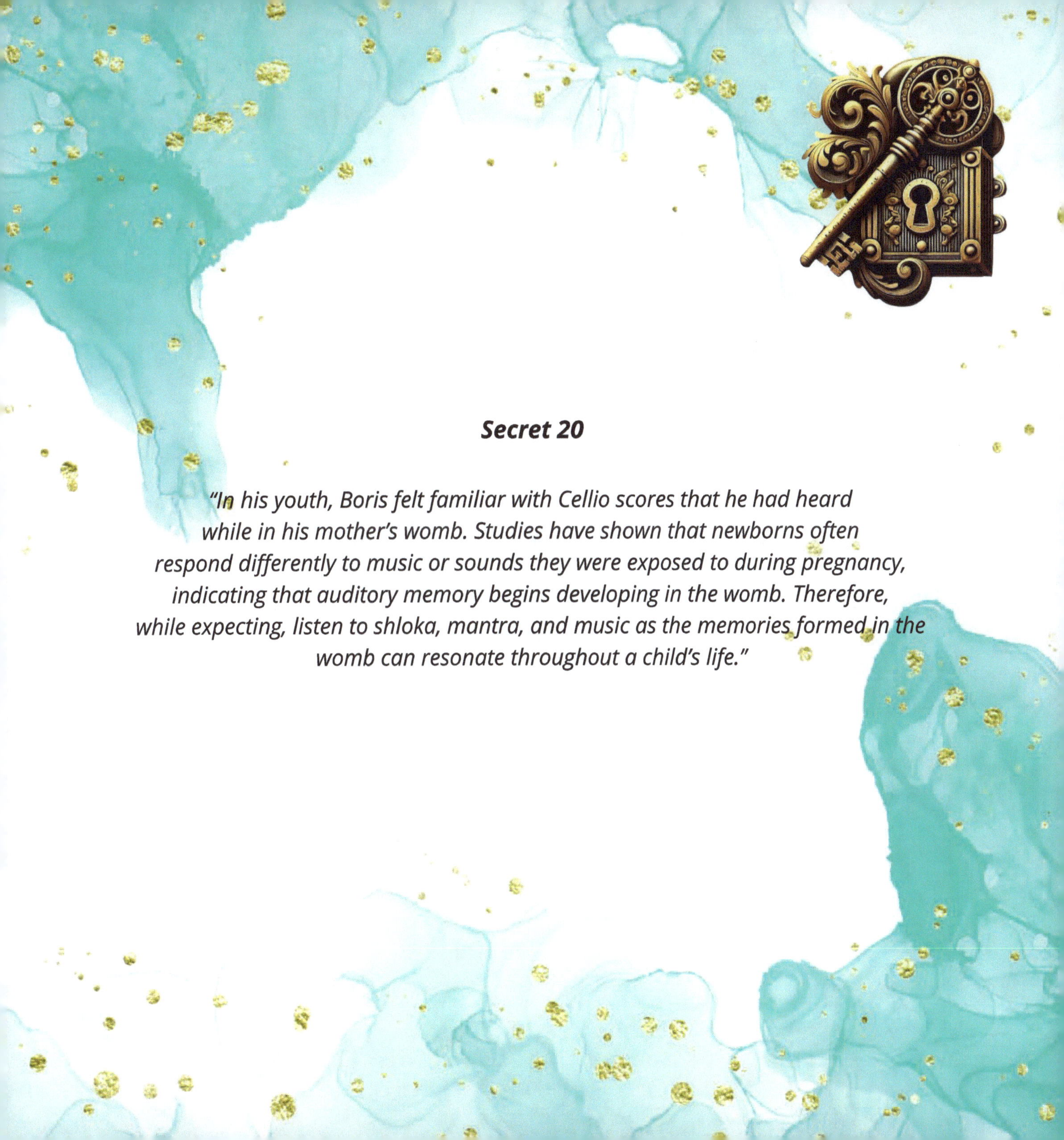

Secret 20

"In his youth, Boris felt familiar with Cellio scores that he had heard while in his mother's womb. Studies have shown that newborns often respond differently to music or sounds they were exposed to during pregnancy, indicating that auditory memory begins developing in the womb. Therefore, while expecting, listen to shloka, mantra, and music as the memories formed in the womb can resonate throughout a child's life."

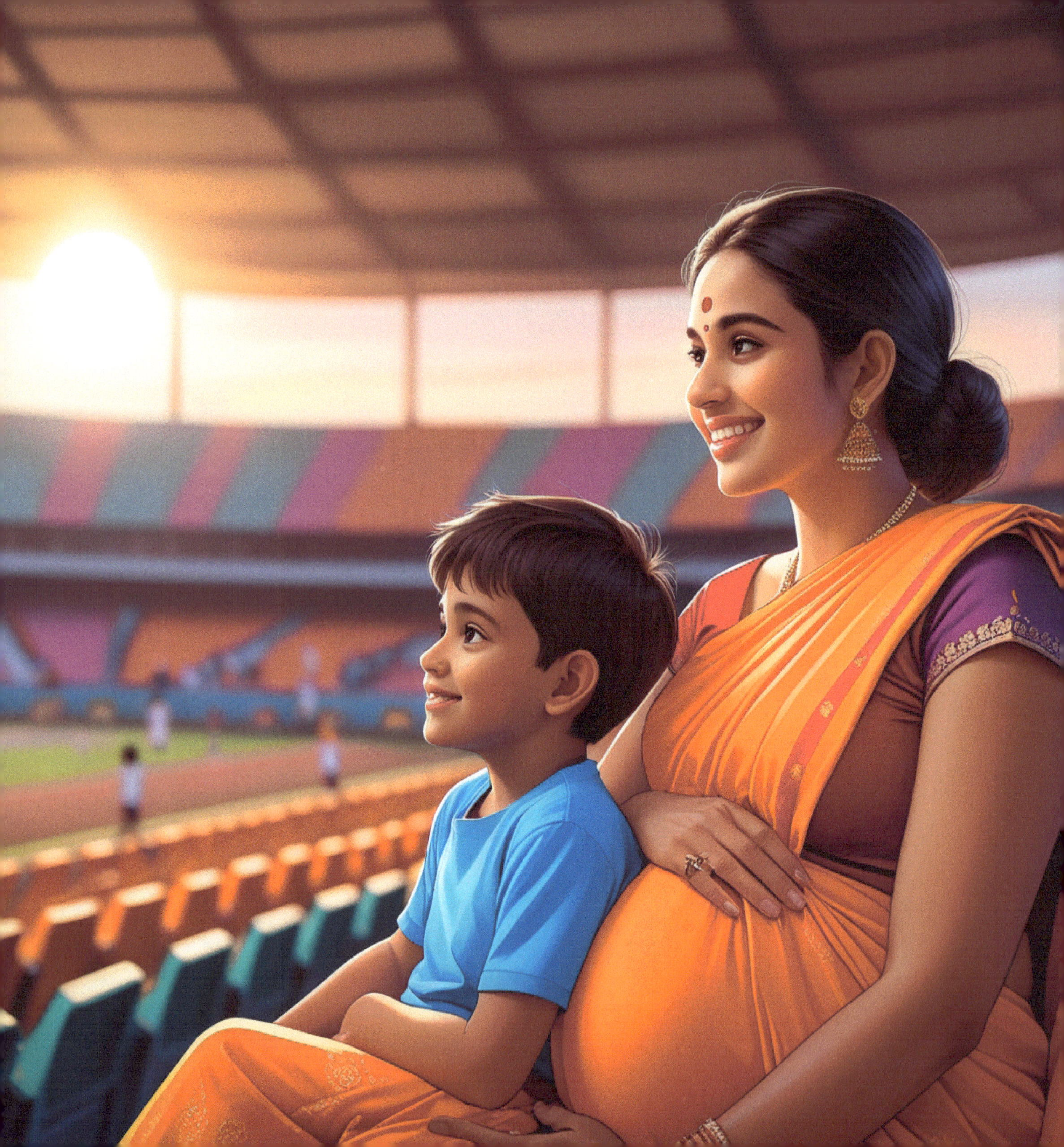

21. The Hidden Influence

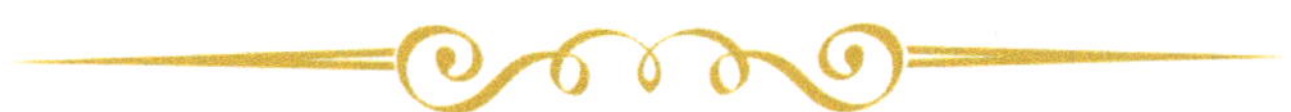

Smita and Shrinivas Mandhana, the proud parents of Smriti Mandhana, always believed in the power of dreams. Smita, a housewife, supported the family at home, while Shrinivas, a chemical distributor by profession, held a deep passion for cricket. Having played at the district level in his younger days, Shrinivas once dreamt of becoming a professional cricketer. However, circumstances prevented him from pursuing it further. He always wished that one of his children would play for India.

Their first child, Shravan, seemed destined to fulfil this wish. From a young age, Shravan was introduced to cricket by his father, and the sport quickly became their shared obsession. Father and son spent hours playing and discussing the game. Four years after Shravan's birth, Smriti was born. When Smriti was 2 years old, the entire family shifted to Sangli from Mumbai. Growing up, Smriti watched her brother play with the same passion, and it was not long before she, too, was captivated by the sport.

Shrinivas never differentiated between his children based on gender and supported Smriti's interest in cricket as well. At just 4 years old, Smriti began accompanying her brother to net practice. As Shravan's talent started gaining attention in local newspapers, Smriti would eagerly cut out clippings for her scrapbook while dreaming of doing the same.

Smriti's journey soon took flight when she began training under coach Anant Tambwekar, a junior state trainer in Sangli. Her talent was undeniable. By the age of 9, she had already made it into the Maharashtra U-15 team, and at 11, she was fast-tracked to the U-19 state team, competing against players much older than her. Smriti's dedication and skill led to her international debut for India at just 16, in a T20 match against Bangladesh.

In June 2018, Smriti was honoured with the BCCI's 'Best Women's International Cricketer' award. Her accolades only grew, with the ICC recognising her with the prestigious Rachael Heyhoe-Flint Award for Women's Cricketer of the Year in 2022, along with many other awards and achievements.

Throughout her journey, Smriti's family remained her strongest support system. To this day, her mother, Smita, takes care of her diet and other personal aspects of her career, while her father manages her cricketing schedule. Although her brother, Shravan, eventually stepped away from cricket, he had a lasting impact on Smriti and often practices with her, encouraging her growth.

When Smriti was asked about her incredible journey and how she achieved such massive success on the reality show Kaun Banega season 15 episode 96 by Amitabh Bachchan, she mentioned, "My father and brother are obsessed with cricket that even from my mom's womb I must have only listened about cricket and only cricket."

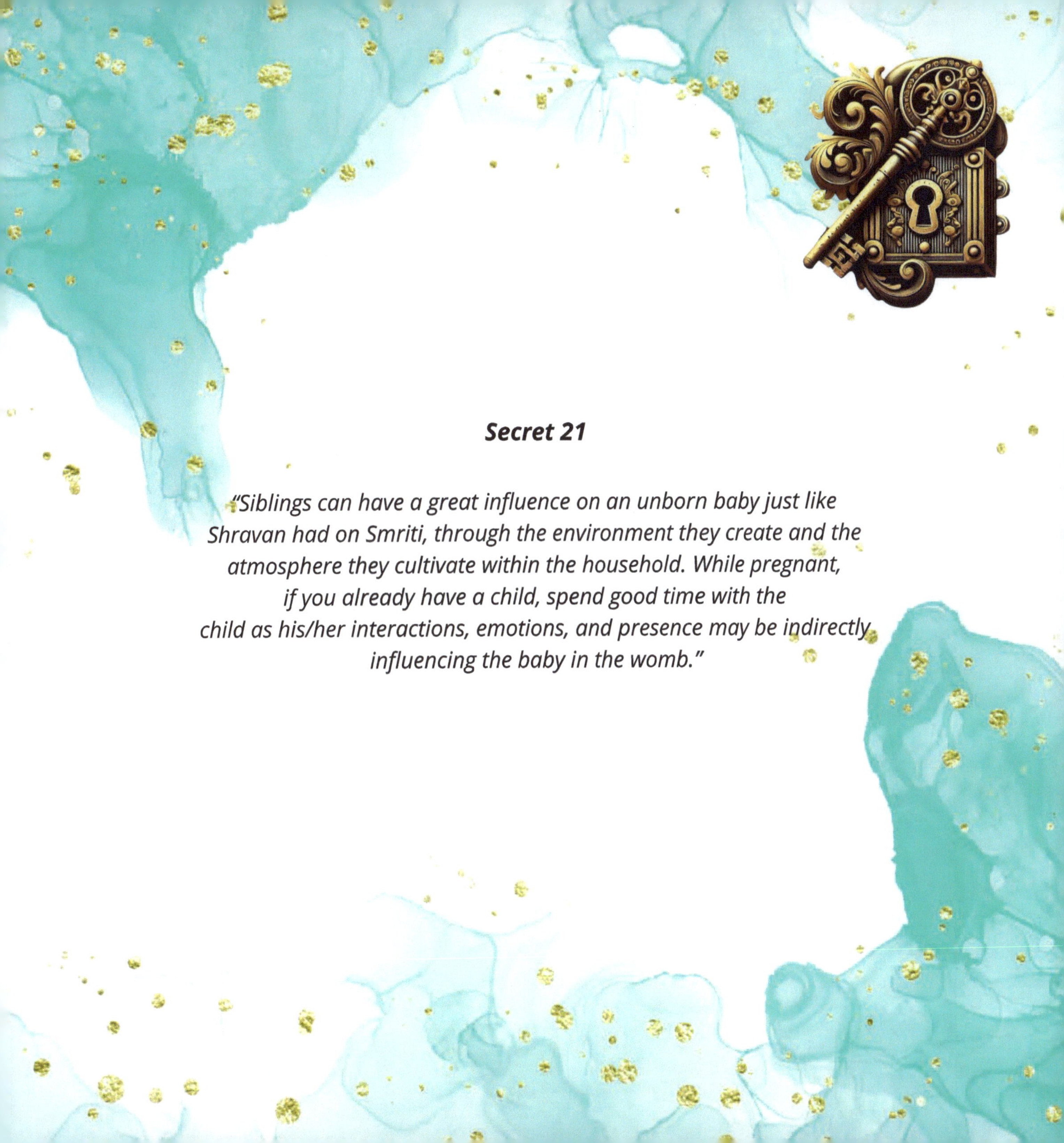

Secret 21

"Siblings can have a great influence on an unborn baby just like Shravan had on Smriti, through the environment they create and the atmosphere they cultivate within the household. While pregnant, if you already have a child, spend good time with the child as his/her interactions, emotions, and presence may be indirectly influencing the baby in the womb."

About Srujan Scientific GarbhSanskar

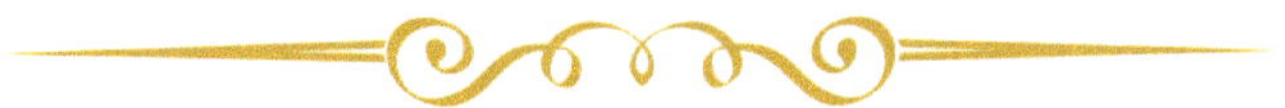

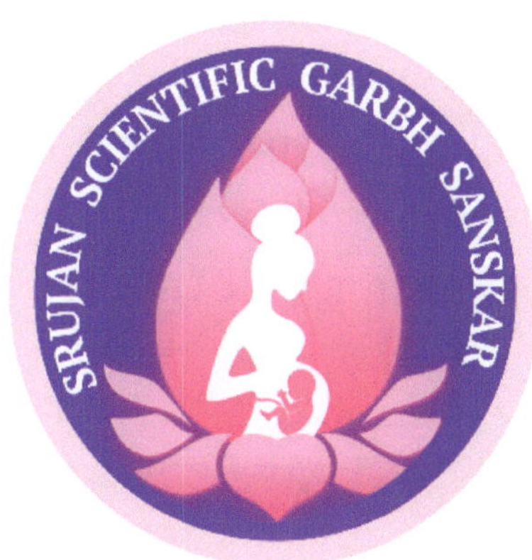

"Where Veda and Vigyana Unite"

Srujan Scientific Garbhsanskar is founded by Er. Payal Mehta, Dr. Pallavi Desai, Dr. Prajakta Gawde with the mission to help 1 million parents bring into this world babies who are physically strong, intellectually genius, emotionally balanced, socially amazing, and spiritually aware. Children are the supreme asset and greatest hope for the future of any nation. If we can have more Swami Vivekananda, Dr. A.P.J. Abdul Kalam and Chhatrapati Shivaji Maharaj, then India leading the world won't be merely a dream.

With over 7 years of experience in GarbhSanskar, Srujan coaches have helped 1000+ parents to have physically, mentally, emotionally, socially, and spiritually fit kids while making their pregnancy journey easy, effortless, joyous, and interesting. Trainers have practised and implemented GarbhSanskar during pregnancy and are "Leading You by Example."

Trainers have a unique way of teaching where they share ancient Vedic secrets in the most scientific and easy-to-implement way.

To know more visit:
Website: https://srujanscientificgarbhsanskar.com
Facebook: https://www.facebook.com/SrujanScientificGarbhasanskar/
Instagram: https://www.instagram.com/srujanscientificgarbhasanskar/
Youtube: https://www.youtube.com/channel/UC0UaJUX9bfpMfNBWaakZ0ZA